Sexuality and Patient Care

Sexuality and Patient Care

A guide for nurses and teachers

Els van Ooijen

and

Andrew Charnock

University of Wales College of Medicine
South East Wales Institute of Nursing and Midwifery Education
Caerleon Education Centre
Gwent
Wales

CHAPMAN & HALL
London · Glasgow · New York · Tokyo · Melbourne · Madras

Published by Chapman & Hall, 2–6 Boundary Row, London SE1 8HN

Chapman & Hall, 2–6 Boundary Row, London SE1 8HN, UK

Blackie Academic & Professional, Wester Cleddens Road,
Bishopbriggs, Glasgow G64 2NZ, UK

Chapman & Hall Inc., One Penn Plaza, 41st Floor, New York
NY 10119, USA

Chapman & Hall Japan, Thomson Publishing Japan, Hirakawacho
Nemoto Building, 6F, 1–7–11 Hirakawa-cho, Chiyoda-ku, Tokyo 102,
Japan

Chapman & Hall Australia, Thomas ˙Nelson Australia, 102 Dodds
Street, South Melbourne, Victoria 3205, Australia

Chapman & Hall India, R. Seshadri, 32 Second Main Road, CIT East,
Madras 600 035, India

Distributed in the USA and Canada by Singular Publishing Group Inc.,
4284 41st Street, San Diego, California 92105

First edition 1994

© 1994 Chapman & Hall

Typeset in 10/12 Palatino by Mews Photosetting, Beckenham, Kent
Printed in Great Britain by St Edmundsbury Press, Bury St Edmunds,
Suffolk

ISBN 0 412 47080 2   1 56593 305 2 (USA)

A catalogue record for this book is available from the British Library

Library of Congress Cataloging-in-Publication data available

∞ Printed on permanent acid-free text paper, manufactured in
accordance with ANSI/NISO Z39.48-1992 and ANSI Z39.48-1984
(Permanence of Paper).

For my father and all the people and friends who have
contributed to my thoughts, ideas and experience
– Els van Ooijen

For Katie and Kieran – Andrew Charnock

Contents

Introduction

There is a growing need for nurses to develop and understand the concept of holistic care. Many of the nursing models in use today acknowledge people as complex beings which include emotional, psychological, social, physical and spiritual dimensions. One dimension is sexuality. Yet there is little material available which helps nurses and other health professionals understand the subject in the context of illness and disability. This book aims to fill a gap in this area of understanding. The style and character of the book are designed to help those who are new to the subject in this context, as well as those who want to extend their knowledge and who have some insight and experience. Various activities have been suggested throughout the book in order to enable learning through discussion. The activities or discussion points can be worked through in groups or, where applicable, individually. It is advisable for teachers to read the chapter about teaching sexuality before using the discussion points contained in the other chapters.

The book has nine chapters, and is designed in such a way that various chapters can be 'dipped into'. This makes the book 'user friendly' which, in the authors' experience, is a prerequisite for understanding an emotive subject.

The chapters follow a logical order. The first chapter offers a brief account of the history of sexuality in different cultures and, as such, places the subject matter into context. It presents in chronological order a picture of how men and women have related to each other, and have been affected by sexuality. Chapter 2 offers a wide definition of sexuality and provides the reader with a framework to explore the various dimensions and perceptions of the subject. It also shows how our understanding of sexuality has changed, and what have been the main influences in such changes. Chapter 3 discusses the ethical and moral problems which surround issues of sexuality (is it any of our business anyway?). A combination of activities and discussions offers the opportunity to discuss possible outcomes of caring for a person's sexual needs in the context of health problems. There are a range of questions and discussion pieces which give the chapter an activity-based format.

The next two chapters, 4 and 5, discuss the ways in which women and men view and experience the world. The style of presentation differs between the two, which reflects their contrasting views. Emphasis is given to potential problems which might arise from those differing perceptions. These chapters have obvious outcomes for those involved in caring for both men and women. Chapter 6 discusses some basic counselling skills, which are further developed in the following chapter. Chapter 7, Sexuality and illness, is written in the format of activities, scenarios and discussion, offering practical suggestions in how to assess and care for people's sexuality.

Chapter 8 contains a range of case studies with questions for the reader and brief model answers. The final chapter is perhaps the most academic. It outlines a detailed plan surrounding the teaching of sexuality. It does this by suggesting a number of discussion points which range in depth and subject matter. It suggests that the teaching of sexuality is best conducted in small workshop or seminar groups, lead by a teacher who is self-aware and informed. This chapter could form the basis of a curriculum model on sexuality. It may also generate ideas for the more casual reader who may be faced with the task of addressing a sexual problem in a clinical context. Throughout the book the authors have presented 'snap shots' of peoples' views and anecdotal accounts from experience. These 'snap shots' are not sub-mitted as definitive, researched pieces: they are offered as a catalyst for further discussion and debate. Many of the activities included in this book have been produced from the authors' work in the areas of sexuality, psychology, counselling and self-awareness.

The book closes with a glossary of both academic and colloquial terms and a list of useful addresses.

CHAPTER 1

The history of sexuality

LEARNING OBJECTIVES

After reading this chapter you should be able to:

1. discuss how the concept of sexuality has changed over a period of time;
2. identify the main features of sexual expression in each of the historical periods identified.

DEVELOPMENT OF SEXUALITY

This section looks at the development of sexuality over a period of time, starting with prehistoric man, up to modern-day expression. Before starting out on this path it may be helpful to answer a significant question. What is a history of sexuality a history of? The answer is somewhat sketchy and disappointing in that it is a history without a proper subject; or as other writers suggest, a history of a subject which is in constant flux (Padgug, 1979; Weeks, 1989). It is probably more to do with preoccupation about the way we live, how we enjoy life, and how we deny or allow physical and emotional pleasures to be fulfilled. The French philosopher (and writer of four volumes on the history of sexuality) Michel Foucault suggests that the concept of sexuality itself is dubious (Foucault, 1979). He goes on to say:

> Sexuality must not be thought of as a kind of natural given force which power tries to hold in check, or as an obscure domain which knowledge tries gradually to uncover. It is the name that can be given to a historical construct (p. 105).

For Foucault, the concept of sexuality is a web of relationships with complex elements; how these elements came together in particular practices might be termed sexuality. The term 'elements' is used to denote notions such as social, cultural and political behaviours. This idea of complex relationships is problematic, because as discussed in

Chapter 2, there are many definitions for sexuality. How, then, does one collect or identify the relevant parts which produce the construct one could call sexuality? And, given such a state of affairs, how trustworthy can a history of sexuality be? The short answer to this is that any history of sexuality must be viewed with a degree of caution. Any attempt to plot the historical course of a subject which is so diverse in its make-up, and which relies on assumptions and suggestions is open to misinterpretation. Consider, for example, one of the definitions given in Chapter 2, that of Gognon and Simons' sociological view, a view which is made up of social interaction, social environment, culture and learned behaviour. If one was to trace these elements back in time, would they have meaning? Would it be easy to suggest how each of the elements related to the concept of sexuality? And does this have a consequence for us today? This last point is even more tenuous. A positive response to these questions would be supported by Mead (1964) and Malinowski (1963), who as social anthropologists recognize the dangers of trying to understand our own previous history by looking at existing societies. The way out is to try and understand each particular society within its own terms of reference. In other words, attempt to live in that era, or see things through their eyes. It is obvious that as one attempts to do this various results will be achieved. Perhaps the mental exercise is more beneficial than the results it sets out to achieve.

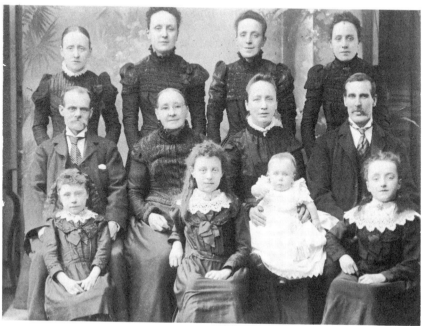

Figure 1.1 A Victorian family.

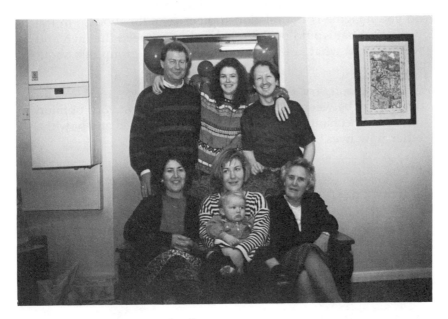

Figure 1.2 A contemporary family.

Figure 1.1 shows a Victorian family, while Figure 1.2 shows a contemporary family. Take a few minutes to reflect on both pictures. Is it possible to imagine what life was like in the Victorian times? Has life changed when one compares it with the twentieth century family in Figure 1.2? Take a moment to look at each of the characters in the pictures, then try activity 1 – family life.

Activity 1: Family life

Take a moment to look at the characters in both of the photographs in Figures 1.1 and 1.2. First, try to imagine how the family in Figure 1.1 lives its life from day to day. Do you imagine that each member may have a particular role? What do you imagine is the relationship between the women in the picture? What would be the relationship between the men and women, and what kind of things would each group talk about socially?

Now take a moment to look at Figure 1.2. Again, try to imagine how the family in Figure 1.2 lives its life from day to day. Do you imagine that each member may have a particular role? What do you imagine is the relationship between the women in the picture? What would be the relationship between the men and women, and what kind of things would each group talk about socially?

On conclusion, try and identify what, if any, are the main differences between each of the families. What in your opinion has caused a change between how one family lived and how the other now lives?

Activity 2 offers an opportunity to discover and discuss some of the major differences that have occurred over a number of generations.

Activity 2: The good old days

Students are asked to talk to a member of their family, for example:

- Father or mother;
- Grandparents;
- Older relatives, aunts, uncles;
- Older member of the community.

The discussion should attempt to discover a number of views using the following questions:

1. What are the major differences between young people today and young people of their generation?
2. How did people socialize?
3. What was the usual way for men and women to meet to start relationships?
4. It is said that in comparison to 20 years ago, we are more promiscuous today. Can they discuss whether this is true?

Students should then form into groups of four and share their results. An attempt is made to correlate the findings and so identify themes and relationships. Each group may then report its findings to the whole group;.

Facilitator's notes (time allowance 90 minutes):

This activity can be carried out within a group setting. It may also be used as individual study projects. *Whichever method is used, there is need to allow time to collect and make sense of the information gathered.*

A variation in the activity could be directed to discovering what has been the main impetus in changes to the above questions.

WHY STUDY THE HISTORY OF SEXUALITY?

Why study the history of sexuality? To understand who we are as adults, we have to have some appreciation of our childhood. Likewise, to comprehend the affect of sexuality in our culture, we need to understand the historical origins. This is not an easy task since we are confronted with the present, mesmerized with the future and neglectful of the past. Hopefully, this chapter will highlight the importance of a historical perception of sexuality on our present-day activities.

What is offered next is a brief historical account of sexuality through the ages, remembering of course to view such accounts with a sceptic, yet open mind. It may also be helpful, after reading the definitions discussed in Chapter 2, to see if certain definitions fit certain periods in our history. However, before entering the realms of history, try the following activity (3).

Activity 3: Sex is ageless

The following are historical periods. For each of them write short notes or statements which could be said to describe sexual expression/behaviour for that particular time.

- Prehistoric;
- Ancient Jews;
- Romans;
- The Middle Ages;
- The Renaissance;
- The Reformation;
- Seventeenth and eighteenth centuries;
- Victorian age;
- Twentieth century.

Facilitator's notes (time allowance 60 minutes):

> *This activity could be carried out by individuals or groups. If done individually, there should be a pooling of ideas, so that themes can be identified, from which discussion can be generated.*
>
> *If used as a group activity, there can be a degree of refinement. For example, each group is given a period in our history. Group members then discuss how sexuality was expressed in that period. Each group then reports back in chronological order under the heading 'Sexuality in our time'. Discussion could also be directed to identifying the sexual role of men and women during a given period.*

IN THE BEGINNING

And the Lord God formed man of the dust of the ground, and breathed into his nostrils the breath of life; and man became a living soul.
  And the man was called Adam.
  And the Lord God caused a deep sleep to fall upon Adam, and he slept: and he took one of his ribs, and closed up the flesh instead thereof. And the rib, which the Lord God had taken from man, made he a woman, and brought her unto the man. And Adam said, this is now bone of my bones, and flesh of my flesh: she shall be called Woman, because she was taken out of man. Therefore shall a man leave his father and mother, and shall cleave unto his wife; and they shall be one flesh. And they were both naked, the man and his wife, and were not ashamed.
Genesis, 2: 7, 21–5

The opening quotes from *The Bible* are probably the earliest literary accounts of man's sexuality. This beginning has even been calculated down to a precise time and date. According to two seventeenth century scholars, Usher and Lightfoot, God created man at nine o'clock in the morning on 23 October (Tannahill, 1980). After the creation in *Genesis, The Bible* then describes the temptation of Adam and Eve, and details the acts of procreation or 'begetting' of various families. For most people, the biblical account is a myth. The evolutionary approach developed by Darwin in *The Descent of Man* (1871) offers a more scientific approach. Darwin's theory relates that over thousands of years, man has developed through a process of selection. This selection has its roots in the animal kingdom, and the types of behaviour carried out by animals. Darwin noted the striking sex differences in both structure and behaviour among many species of animals. He observed that males were larger, stronger and more aggressive. Males would take the initiative in courting and would often fight to defend their claim to females.

This type of behaviour is still very much in evidence in our culture today. Visit any disco or pub and you will see how people attempt to develop and maintain relationships with the opposite sex. The degree of success of such relationships is often a fraught affair, as any young person will testify. The success and bravado at such situations seem to be in direct proportion to the amount of alcohol consumed, something our animal ancestors did not have to contend with.

Activity 4: What's a nice girl like you ... ?

The participants are invited to discuss or role-play one or any number of the following scenarios. The purpose of this activity is to raise awareness to types of sexual behaviour. It may also identify colloquial vocabulary.

Scenario 1

You are out at a disco with a group of girl or boy friends. At the bar you notice a good looking woman/man who appears to be 'giving you the eye'. What's your next move? What sort of things would you say?

Scenario 2

Every day at the bus stop you meet this man/woman. You smile at each other and exchange good mornings, but that is all. You would like to get to know him/her a little more; how would you go about this?

Scenario 3

You are out with the 'lads' one night and being slightly worse the wear from the affects of alcohol, you attempt to chat up a girl. What would you say? What would her response be?

Scenario 4

You are out with a group of women for the evening when the subject of men's chat-up lines comes up in conversation. Each of you then take it in turn to list the types of chat-up lines you have had.

Facilitator's notes (time allowance 90 minutes):

The activity is to be carried out in small groups of no more than six people. The opportunity for individuals to 'pass' on the activity must be allowed. The group members are given the above scenarios, which after discussion they could either discuss or role-play particular one/s to the rest of the group.

PREHISTORIC

Prehistoric man (or woman; one supposes there is no way of knowing) were great painters of what they saw around them. It is from these paintings that our knowledge of sexuality is taken. Paintings in prehistoric times show males and females in sexual poses even to the point of sexual intercourse. There seems to have been magical qualities attached to the sex act, a feature often depicted in the paintings.

One of the commonly held notions of Stone Age man and his sexual behaviour is the image of him dragging 'his' woman off by the hair, presumably 'to have his way with her'. However, this idea has little or no foundation in fact. What the cave paintings suggest is that sexual expression and behaviour at the time may have been violent. This serves as a reminder of the basic, almost animal instinct (see Freud) lurking beneath our calm exteriors, an instinct that is kept in check by social and cultural pressures, as we conform to expected patterns of behaviour. Yet on occasions the animal instinct can break through and wreak havoc on an unsuspecting society. The all-too-familiar violent and outrageous sexual acts (rape or child abuse) are extreme examples of such behaviour.

Prehistoric man, it would appear, did not confine his artistic flair simply to cave paintings. The Venus figurine (Figure 1.3), of which 60 or more have been found in various parts of central Europe, stands about five inches tall, and is usually made out of ivory, clay or

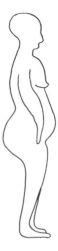

Figure 1.3 Venus figurine.

soft stone. The Venuses are sculptures of feminine form, with the maternal parts grossly distorted. Opinions on the role and function of these statues differ, with suggestions ranging from 'sexual', 'magical call on fertility', to 'religious', or 'non-religious'. Whatever the reason for creating such an image, one fact is unmistakable, man was beginning to take notice and to examine his mate.

EGYPTIAN

In the ancient East, relationships with the supernatural, sex and fertility were very evident. In Egypt, fertility cults existed, and sexual symbolism was a crucial ingredient in most religious practices, with phallic icons being very visible. Intercourse with a virgin, who was ritualistically 'deflowered', was of great importance (an idea that still holds true today). Prostitution, both male and female, was performed in temples. Heterosexual, homosexual and oral–genital activity was also apparent. Despite this somewhat promiscuous state of affairs, laws against adultery are some of the oldest moral laws.

The position of women in Egypt was one of underlings. The daughter was the property of the father during childhood, and of her husband in married life. The prime purpose of taking a wife was to bear children and to keep house, a type of 'upper servant'. Marriage could take place early in the girl's life; marriage at the age of 11 or 12 was not uncommon. The birth of a son for the husband was of paramount importance. Pregnancy testing of 4000 years ago was commonplace, as it is today. However, the techniques have changed. Egyptian doctors wrapped two separate cloth parcels, one containing wheat, the other barley. The pregnant woman was told to urinate on the parcels every day. If both parcels sprouted she would give birth. If the wheat sprouted first it would be a boy; if the barley sprouted first, then a girl would be born. Wheat was a much more valued grain than barley!

ANCIENT JEWS

Ancient Jews, in contrast to other societies living in the Near East, were quite inflexible in their outlook on sex. Masturbation was considered a means of contraception, while celibacy was considered a sin. Other activities which led to non-procreation were also forbidden. The sexual act was for the procreation of children only, a factor that was positively reinforced. For example, a newly married man was free from military and work obligations for a number of months, presumably to start a family right away. This practice can still be seen in today's society – the so-called 'honeymoon period' after marriage. The Judaic way of life was recorded in the *Old Testament* of *The Bible* and was treated as a guide to living. Many sexual practices were outlawed; homosexuality, incest and adultery were prohibited. The act of masturbation by men was also forbidden as it wasted the seeds of reproduction. Sexual relations were for the production of children, anything that fell outside this was considered immoral. Women were considered inferior to men. Men were allowed to own property. The inheritance of such property was to be passed on to sons, and hence the need for male offspring. There were unusual purification periods after the birth of children. A woman required 33 days to purify herself if a son was born, but 55 days before she could engage in sexual intercourse if a daughter was born.

ANCIENT GREEKS

There is no greater nor keener pleasure than that of bodily love – and none which is more irrational.

Plato

The Greek civilization produced the first common patterns of what may be considered moral sexual behaviour. Greek culture was plagued with the idea of pleasing, and adhering to what the Gods considered correct behaviour for mortals. Sex and beauty were considered important values. During this time various Greek stories and myths were created which described the fears and phenomena of sexual activities. The legend of Oedipus, who, without knowing it, murders his father and marries his mother, was later interpreted by Freud as a sign of a young male's desire to take the place of the father and possess the mother; to this day it is referred to as the Oedipus complex (Freud, 1905). Other Grecian fables indicate an awareness of immodesty. Narcissus loved himself so much that he could not love another.

The Greeks in their art and literature depicted all types of sexual activity. Sexual intercourse was portrayed in a variety of positions. Fellation was presented as the norm, probably taking place before intercourse. The whole of the sexual act was a joyful event. Diversion from the so-called norm was acceptable, as long as it did not replace heterosexual activity; bisexuality was commonplace. Men were allowed to have sexual relations outside the marriage. Such freedom permitted the use of prostitutes and slaves within the household. The Greeks considered both men and women to be bisexual; therefore, homosexuality was accepted and widely practised, more so among men and boys than among females. Sexual involvement between men and boys (pederasty) was considered as part of the boys' development, contributing to the intellectual and passionate growth in the boy. Men who engaged in homosexual activities were also married and were able to fulfil the responsibility of family life, that is, to produce large families.

The position of women was inferior to men in Greek society. The woman had two principal roles – as a wife running the home, and as the bearer of children. Female homosexuality was not assigned much importance. However, it is from the Greek female poet Sappho, who lived with other women on the island of Lesbos, that the term lesbianism is derived.

ROMANS

The main difference between Greek sexuality and Roman sexuality was that the Romans viewed sex in more physical terms. The body was appreciated more as a sexual instrument rather than a carrier of passion and emotions. The infamous Roman games stand as testimony to this point. While Greek society attempted to extol the virtues of homosexuality, the Romans viewed it as part of sexual life. Other accepted forms of sexual behaviour were pederasty, oral intercourse and transvestism.

The sexual culture of Romans is still very much in evidence today. A trip to the old city of Pompeii reveals explicit insight in to a society's sexual exploits. The Romans were very business-like about their sexuality. Pompeii is littered with murals, effigies and sculptures depicting sexual appreciation. On a number of the roadways are chiselled impressions of male genitals which point the would-be client in the direction of the house where prostitutes could be found. In some instances an erect phallic symbol could be found above the door of a prostitute's house, the projection being clearly visible from the end of the street. Phallic symbols were endowed with magical powers. Representations of the penis, large and small, were found as charms around the neck, while others could be found over homes, shops and city gates. The idea behind displaying such an object was to ward off evil spirits, whose gaze would be deflected when it fell upon the phallus.

THE MIDDLE AGES

In the period of the Middle Ages, which is the period from the fall of the Roman Empire until the Renaissance, the Catholic church was the mainstay of ideals and philosophies regarding sexual activities. Forming the predominant ways of thinking during this time were the concepts of virtue, compassion, love, chastity and abstinence. Intercourse was viewed only as a means of procreation, and only to be enjoyed by married couples. Married couples were even advised about the preferred positions for intercourse. Many pious couples would have intercourse wearing a heavy nightshirt with a hole cut out to allow penetration. Wearing such clothes prevented other intimate body contact. Intercourse was to take place with the man in the dominant position, other positions could be met by severe penance. On certain days of the week, couples were urged not to have intercourse. Days for abstaining were: Thursdays, which was in memory of the arrest of Jesus, Fridays, in commemoration of his death; Saturdays, in honour of the blessed Virgin Mary; Sunday was the day of resurrection; and Mondays, in honour of the faithful who died (Tannahill, 1980).

Methods of contraception and abortion were forbidden. As for 'deviant' behaviour, homosexuality was punishable by death. Although this appears a harsh time for any form of sexual freedom, the majority of the people paid only lip service to such high ideals. Much of eroticism was driven underground, and emerged in the most unlikely of places. Decorations on churches, on choir stalls and religious sculptures of the time show provocative poses of both males and females, even to the point of men with erections and couples engaged in sexual intercourse. Moreover, some Irish churches have carved effigies of genital symbols which were thought to be protection against evil (possibly a continuance of the Roman ideas).

Women in the Middle Ages were held in low esteem, and their purpose in life was to bear sons. The nobility of the time could use the women of the lower social class for sexual purposes without redress.

THE RENAISSANCE AND REFORMATION

This was a time when art and literature became important ideals. Many of the older views of sexual freedom and enjoyment became popular again. Artists painted the human body in various erotic poses. Laws against deviant behaviours were constructed mainly to protect the young. The Renaissance was a time when sexuality was seen as exuberant. Immense wealth coupled with desire and luxury led the ruling classes to overindulge in sexual exploits. It was open season on women. Prostitutes could practise without recrimination; this was until syphilis appeared in the sixteenth century, which dramatically curtailed prostitutes' activities, and the regulation of brothels began (Hyam, 1991). Again, as with most historical eras, women were treated as inferior to men.

The Reformation, as the title suggests, was a period in the sixteenth century where reform of political, social and, more importantly, religious affairs took place. There was in short a reaction to the Renaissance period of life. The Roman Catholic church lost importance, while the Protestant churches developed their sphere of influence.

This lead to a specific almost official change in Christian teaching about sexual activity. There appear to be two main characters who were effective in bringing about change – Martin Luther and John Calvin. Martin Luther's views on sex and marriage was much more down-to-earth than the Catholic perspective. Luther rejected the view that marriage was sacrosanct, mainly because he could find no biblical support for this point of view. This led him to suggest that marriage had a more erotic element, and that sexual urges were part of God's will, and there was no point in suppressing such feelings. He compared marriage to a hospital that cured one of lust and avoided fornication (Feucht, 1961). Where a marriage failed to fulfil the sexual needs, it lost its main purpose for its existence, a situation which could be grounds for divorce.

John Calvin, another leader in the Reformation, did not agree with Luther's view that marriage was a remedy for sin. Instead, Calvin observed marriage to be a veil which covered sin. Calvinism suggests that a husband should humble himself before his wife and approach her with delicacy and propriety. This mentality extended to a disapproving of most things frivolous and ebullient.

SEVENTEENTH AND EIGHTEENTH CENTURIES

This period in our history has been referred to as the 'age of reason', primarily because it was the age of scientific discoveries – Galileo, Newton and Descartes were all prominent in providing scientific answers to nature's mysteries. This meant that *The Bible* decreased in importance as the solver of life's complexities. The enigma of sex decreased and a more 'laid back' approach to sexual matters was adopted. During this Elizabethan period, sex was an activity to be laughed at, written about or even performed, as evident in many of Shakespeare's plays.

Things did not stay like this for long; the revolution of Oliver Cromwell in 1649 saw the establishment of Puritanism. This effectively condemned sexual expression of any kind, even in marriage: sex was considered only for procreation. As we have seen in previous eras such a 'clamp down' on sexual freedom leads to periods of licentious and immoral behaviour. Such was the case with the restoration of the monarchy of King Charles the Second. Sensuality, promiscuity and sexual mayhem became evident. Adultery and scandal appeared to increase people's social standing rather than reduce it. The recent film *Dangerous Liaisons* conjures up and depicts this type of sexual disorder. It must be remembered that around this time explorers were investigating new worlds and civilizations, and in some cases bringing back elements of the culture visited (for example, Cook's visit to Tahiti in 1771).

Later, in the eighteenth century, attitudes towards sexuality changed again, and tolerance gave way to inhibition. The Methodist movement, led by John Wesley, denounced man's flagrant use of sexuality. Men and women became discreet in their private and sexual lives. So the next century dawned with sexual expression under tight restraint; enter the Victorian age.

VICTORIAN AGE

England has always been disinclined to accept human nature.
E.M. Forster, 1987, p. 196

The Victorian age, so-named after the reign of Queen Victoria from 1837 to 1901, is an era which is possibly one of the most talked about, written about and effective aspects of our sexual history. The foundations laid in this period about what was acceptable sexual behaviour still have repercussions on today's society. The material on sexuality in this age is excessive to the point that it becomes overwhelming. What is offered here is a discussion of the major themes occurring in this epoch.

Suppression and denial are key descriptive words in any debate of the Victorian period. Major forces for controlling sexuality were the preservation and sanctity of the home and the family. The wife's responsibility was to look after the home and the needs of her husband. Men were urged to marry late, the usual age being 30. The ideal woman for marriage would be pure, in every sense of the word: she would be a virgin, and be unable to have or display sexual feelings. She was also delicate, quiet and submissive. If women did display sexual feelings, or found the sexual act pleasurable, they were considered to have a 'problem'. An eminent London urologist of the time, William Acton, would solve this problem by surgically removing the clitoris (a clitoridectomy). Some Victorian women unfortunately suffered this because they, their husbands or their physicians were greatly disturbed by their natural sexual response and desire (Godow, 1982). Women were very much objects of men's desires.

For the men who chose to marry late it was acceptable behaviour for them to satisfy their sexual urges with prostitutes or the lower social classes.

To protect the innocence of women and children, reference to anything sexual was prohibited. Books, medical and scientific journals were suppressed or closely censored. Literary censorship and suppression were practised with amazing zeal. The novelist Thomas Hardy seemed to be inflicted with more than his fair share of censorship. When he first submitted his manuscript of *Tess of the D'Urbervilles* in 1889, it was returned to him on the grounds that although the publishers were aware that such tragedies were happening, it would be advisable not to publicise it in case notoriety increased acceptability. Hardy then became adept at preparing and censoring his own work. Sometimes the changes Hardy was asked to make were minimal. In *The Trumpet Major*, for example, he was advised to change a lover's meeting from Sunday to a Saturday. Other changes were verging on the ridiculous. When *Jude the Obscure* first appeared, the word 'couch' was substituted for 'bed', 'sex' was changed to 'affection', and 'kissing' was replaced by 'shaking hands'. The trials and tribulations in the publication (or not) of *Lady Chatterley's Lover* by D.H. Lawrence is another case which adequately depicts the traumas faced by those writers who to all intents and purposes were just telling the truth. Oscar Wilde was another Victorian writer who, because of his flair both on and off the written page, suffered dearly for his outlandish escapades.

The environment and conversation were also to be protected from sexual expression (piano legs had to be draped so as not to conjure up thoughts of human legs, and what that might lead to). The decorative appearance of many Victorian homes was large, dark and formal. Many of the sofas produced were designed in an 'S' or 'U' shape so that people could not touch or sit close together; because of this they became known as 'unsociables'.

Windows were heavily draped, often with the addition of wooden shutters. Many of the houses had ornate ironwork fencing around them, adding to the privacy demanded within the home. It is not hard to imagine that such sombre decorative features were reflective of the sexual mood of the age.

In conversation, words such as breasts, hips and buttocks were discouraged from common usage. Some words were not discouraged but merely changed for less harsh and vulgar ones. For instance, 'whore' became 'fallen woman', masturbation was replaced with 'self-abuse'. No-one at the dinner table was allowed to ask for a thigh, breast or leg of meat. If anyone was to mention inappropriate or suggestive words which caused ladies to swoon, then smelling salts would always be on hand to aid recovery.

The Victorian age is synonymous with the concept of Empire. Hyam (1991) has performed a detailed critique of the effect of people and their sexuality in the building and development of the British Empire.

His book, *Empire and Sexuality: The British Experience*, calls into question many of the sexual persuasions and activities of the people who helped build and develop the British Empire. The activities and persuasions of Gordon, Kitchener, Montgomery and even Churchill are examined, with fascinating insight. For example, Hyam highlights the exploits of Robert Baden-Powell, founder of the Boy Scout Movement. Baden-Powell, who had an asexual relationship with his wife, was deeply fearful of any female sexuality. This led to a transference of sexual interests to a life-long fascination with the male sex, especially boys. To quote Hyam: 'The Scout Movement was the creative offspring, at once cathartic and narcissistic, of these sexual tensions' (p. 41). In simple terms, the Scout movement was developed to satisfy a sexual need. This demonstrates just one of a number of people who have been, or who are, influenced by their sexuality, an influence that has affected many institutions, and still may do so today.

In summary, what we appear to have is a society that is very repressive, dogmatic, arrogant and puritanical. But was this the case? There is some evidence to suggest that although on the surface most activities were tightly controlled, there was an underlying, almost black-market activity surrounding sexual conduct. Or as Humphries puts it, *A Secret World of Sex* (1988). Humphries' book was made into a compelling television series, based on many first-hand accounts of the treatment of sexuality between 1900 and 1950. With words and striking illustrations, Humphries moves the reader through personal histories in which people suffered greatly for the sake, or mistake, of sexual expression.

THE SECRET WORLD OF SEX

There is extensive literature on Victorian sexuality, especially on those things people wished to keep secret. The discussion here centres around prostitution, its incidence, and contributing factors which lead people to take up what some have called the 'oldest profession'.

Throughout Victorian Britain, prostitution was rife. By the mid-nineteenth century there were more brothels than schools. These brothels were not confined just to London; it was possible to find a prostitute in most regions in Britain. Police estimates of known prostitutes in London were of around 5000 to 7000 between 1858 and 1868. For the country as a whole, the approximate number of prostitutes was between 24 000 and 30 000. These figures do not include the incalculable number of unknown prostitution; one author suggests the total number (which includes known and unknown) to be around 80 000 (Hyam, 1991). These are staggering statistics in an age of so-called high moral standing.

There has been some debate as to the cause of female prostitution. Some reasons have been listed as follows.

1. Social necessity, a means of making a living in hard times. This view is somewhat devalued when it is seen that the majority of women who turn to prostitution come from a domestic service background, a group at this time who were free from financial anxieties. An analysis of over 3700 prostitutes carried out in the early part of the century by the Chaplain of Clerkenwell Women's Prison suggests that for more than half these women, the main cause of turning to prostitution was being lead astray by other girls.
2. The lure of prostitution (Gay, 1986), that is the general attraction to the 'seedier' side of life – being taken out for the evening by a young gentleman, wined and dined for favour of sexual pleasures.
3. Demand must also have been a contributing factor to the rise in prostitution. As stated earlier, there was a shortage of willing sex partners because of the restraint women were under, and the fact that men were expected to marry late. It is easy to see that in such a state of affairs, prostitution arose out of sexual frustration. This idea is said to be supported by the decline in prostitution in about 1918 as increasingly compliant girlfriends, protected by contraception, gave way to the demands of boyfriends (Hyam, 1991).

Prostitution was not confined simply to females; male prostitution was also prevalent, but seldom discussed. It is suggested that there were a small number of brothels specializing in men and boys in London. The military was also noted for attracting those whose propensities were to indulge in homosexual activities. A well-established male brothel was located near the barracks in Regent's Park (Chesney, 1970).

THE VOICE OF REASON

Havelock Ellis (1859–1939)

This discourse paints a dull, unenlightened picture (that is, if we compare it to today's attitudes) of people's attitudes towards sexuality. It is worth noting at this point that in all of this suppression and undercover activity concerning sexual expression, there was one writer who appeared to express some rational ideas. No discussion on Victorian sexuality would be complete without mentioning the ideas of the physician Havelock Ellis (1859–1939). His work shows interesting insight, especially as it pre-dates the research findings of Kisney *et al.* (1948, 1953), Masters and Johnson (1966), and others whose work followed some several years later.

Ellis came from a strict Victorian home full of the sexually repressive attitudes of the time. This interest in sexuality developed as a result of personal problems. As a young man he suffered from nocturnal emissions. Aware of the possible consequences of such actions – disease, blindness, insanity, acne, even death – his curiosity developed into a life-long quest of attempting to understand the workings of his own and other people's sexuality. Thereafter, Ellis spent several years studying and writing about human sexuality. Although much of his work is illuminating, what remains impressive (for his time) is his 'naturalistic non-judgemental' view of human sexuality. This is evident in his writings:

> *The sexual impulse is a force, to some extent an incalculable force, and the struggle of the man to direct that force, when he and it are both constantly changing, is inevitably attended with peril (p. 305).*

Ellis is best known for his book entitled *Studies in the Psychology of Sex* (1933). Much of the material for his writings was gathered from his own knowledge about sexuality, medical literature, anthropological studies and case histories from his patients. A synopsis of his findings is as follows.

1. The act of masturbation is common among females and males.
2. There are varying degrees of heterosexuality and homosexuality.
3. Sexual problems are more often psychological than physiological.
4. Sexual behaviour starts at an early age and continues throughout the age range.
5. The sexual appetite of Victorian women is pure fiction.
6. Orgasm in males and females is similar.
7. Women often experience multiple orgasm.

Ellis was of the belief that sexuality was a very variable concept, not only among individuals but across cultures and societies. This idea is important when attempting to understand and assess various forms of sexual expression. Human beings tend to generalize and stereotype behaviours and attitudes. They do this by working from the belief that one's own personal experience is similar to everyone else's. Such an idea is supported by the discussions in Chapter 2 on definitions of sexuality. It is becoming more and more difficult to have a clear-cut distinction between 'normal' sexuality and 'abnormal' sexuality.

Ellis found from his case studies and personal correspondence that many people had suffered as a consequence of ignorance and suppression of their sexuality. This affected him deeply, so much so that he became a staunch activist for reform and positive sex education. Some of Ellis's ideas may still appear a little extreme even by today's standards. For example, Ellis advocated: early sex education for boys and girls, an idea that has recently been reborn ('Sex education should start at five, say MPs', *Independent Newspaper*, 7 November, 1991); acceptance of sexual behaviour in young children as a form of development and self-exploration; sexual experimentation for young couples before marriage; equal rights for women, especially in the area of divorce and contraception; the right to private sexual behaviour by consenting adults of the same sex. It is easy to see how such suggested reforms and ideas would be treated as abominable by the Victorians of the time. However, how well do the above notions sit within today's society? Are there still taboo areas?

Sigmund Freud (1856–1939)

Dying in the same year as Ellis, Sigmund Freud (1856–1939) was another prolific writer on the subject of sexuality. Through his work with patients (most of whom were women) suffering from mental disorders, Freud developed theories about personality, human development and character. His ideas and writing have greatly influenced society's thinking and understanding about how people function psychologically. Part of Freud's work looked at the subject of sexuality. He wrote three essays on the theory of sexuality and other works (Freud, 1905). While Freud's work was highly theoretical, and therefore difficult to prove or disprove, his contribution has none-the-less added greatly to our understanding of human sexuality.

The subject of sexuality and sexual pleasure was a central theme in Freud's view of human life. He believed that people were motivated by the desire for pleasure, and the avoidance of pain. The concept of pleasure for Freud always had a sexual meaning. This he explained was not pleasure derived from genital stimulation, but from gratification in a broader sense – well-being, relationships, attainment and a sense of belonging. Consider this point for a moment, and then look at activity 5.

Activity 5: Pleasure

Take a few minutes to make a list of activities, behaviours and attitudes, that give you pleasure, make you happy or you enjoy doing.

Are you able to identify any sexual connections or connotations from the list that you have made?

The driving force behind seeking pleasure Freud termed 'libido', or sex drive. Libido was seen as a form of energy, that is, the psychological representation of a biological force. The force of libido would, and needed to, have a form of expression. It is impossible, Freud argued, to suppress libido energy since it will find an avenue of expression in some form. A controversial aspect of Freud's libido energy was that it was present from birth. He proposed that during the first year of life a baby's sucking instinct was the result of libido, or sexual urge. The satisfaction and contentment following infant feeding is a precursor of feelings for sexual satisfaction later in life.

Sexual urges or feelings can be manifested in other parts of the body. It is as if our sexual impulses have to find an outlet or discharge point. Freud believed that libido force could be channelled to various points in the body, essentially where there was a collection of nerve fibres, for example, the mouth. These so-called erogenous zones would change location as they moved through a developmental excitatory phase. So from birth the mouth would be the primary area, moving to the anus, and ending finally with the genitalia. To develop successfully, in a sexual sense, Freud postulated that humans had to move through each of the stages to be psychosexually well-adjusted. These theories are the mainstay of Freud's explanation of any sexual problems that may become manifest. If, for example, a child has problems at any one of the psychosexual 'milestones', this could create problems resulting in perversion or inversion (Freud's words).

This brief outline of Freud's theories has been detailed so that the historical impact is noted. More than any other writer, Freud has affected our understanding, explanation and sometimes treatment of psychosexual problems. He believed that sex was instinctive and that it should be expressed by appropriate channels. Too tight a control on sexual expression could lead to psychological and sexual problems being expressed unhealthily, he stated. Regardless of whether one accepts Freud's theories about the origins and nature of sexuality, he has been a major force in expressing the virtue of natural sexual expression. This later point (natural sexual expression) could well be a fitting description of present-day behaviour.

PRESENT DAY

The twentieth century has seen many changes within the concept of human sexuality. As a whole, the trend has been for more sexual freedom. Certainly, 30 years ago it would have been unthinkable to consider writing a book of this nature. There has been an increase in the gathering of objective data on sexuality, the work of Masters and Johnson in the 1970s is a case in point. However, it would be wrong to suggest that all people today are totally sexually aware or self-actualized. To some extent, old views and values still impinge on our daily lives. Consider the following questions. Is there a disparity between what young and old discuss about aspects of sexuality? Is the exposure and nature of varying forms of sexual expression an issue young and old agree on? The likely answers to these and many other issues cause a restraining influence on sexual behaviour and expression. Before moving on to analyse the major contributing factors which have affected sexuality, try the following activity (6).

Activity 6: A sign of the times

For each of the following dates and topic areas identify what major changes have taken place.

Topic Area:	Science	Marriage	Religion	Media
Year				
1950				
1960				
1970				
1980				
1990				
2000				

Facilitator's notes (time allowance 1.5 hours):

The participants are invited to work in small groups. Once the activity has been completed, the group reforms. A master grid should be developed which shows all the material generated by the individual groups.

As a variation, the topic areas could be changed. For example, politics, position of women in society, travel, education, work, industrialization and fashion.

There has been an unmistakable growth and development in science and technology. The treatment of venereal disease and the development of contraceptive devices and techniques (for example, the Femidom for women) have contributed to a liberation of sexual attitudes and behaviour. However, the recent human immuno-deficiency virus (HIV) and acquired immune deficiency syndrome (AIDS) epidemics may have affected sexual behaviour, or have they? In the work being carried out at the moment on sexual lifestyles and HIV risk, there has been no appreciable decrease in sexual activity (Johnson *et al.*, 1992). Research by Francome (1979) shows an increase in both male and female sexual intercourse (Table 1.1).

Table 1.1 Experience of sexual intercourse

Males with experience of sexual intercourse				Females with experience of sexual intercourse		
Age	1964	1975		Age	1965	1975
16	14%	32%		16	5%	21%
17	26%	50%		17	10%	37%
18	34%	65%		18	17%	47%

(After: Francome, 1979.)

The increase in medical treatment has led to a reduction of fears about unwanted pregnancy. Even the 'morning-after' contraceptive pill allows for greater liberalization of sexual activity. The growth in scientific knowledge has been mirrored by a decline in religious beliefs and attitudes towards sexuality. The various denominations appear to have weakened their resolve in disposition to sexual behaviour. The recent agreement by the church to allow the ordination of women, although primarily a gender issue, is none-the-less related to sexuality. The revelations of a Catholic priest having an illegitimate son must have repercussions on the spiritual respectability and credibility of the church.

The development of inner city areas with the concomitant reduction in rural living has led to a more impersonal and over-populated environment. Such an environment has the potential to present more opportunities for sexual encounters. The increase in anonymity, together with a decrease in close-knit community life, may be synonymous with a growth in sexual expression and behaviour. The population is now much more mobile, allowing people to move freely around the country. The availability of transport has greatly affected the mobility of society. It is now possible to fly to countless areas in the world. Even personal transportation has become readily accessible, thus providing privacy, especially to the younger age group. The potential to use the vehicle for sexual exploits is often the butt of many jokes – the 'passion wagon'!

The media must also figure largely in any debate of sexuality in the twentieth century. All forms of media expression have played a part in raising society's awareness of sexuality. Television, radio, films, literature and newspapers provide an opportunity for discussion and focusing on sexuality. It is impossible nowadays to watch television or read a daily newspaper without identifying a sexual theme or issue. The clothing industry has also had its fair share of sexual expression. Many fashion crazes today have a statment to make about the person and the culture in which we live.

Feminism or the women's movement, which started in the nineteenth century with the suffragettes, has seen a recent revival. The position of women in society has changed drastically, especially when compared to the Victorian era. The liberation of women in employment, the home and relationships has influenced the sexual views and attitudes of our society. The women's movement advocates equal rights in all areas of life – for example, social, political and sexual rights. Some achievements have been obvious, for example, Margaret Thatcher became the first woman prime minister. Nevertheless, inequality of some thousands of years is not easily remedied, and old-style beliefs and values still remain. The majority of top industrial, business and government positions are still held by men.

Activity 7: Famous names

Make a list of famous people who fit the following categories:

- Sport ....
- Entertainment ....
- Politics ....
- Authors ....
- Medicine ....
- Journalism ....
- Art ....
- Architecture ....

After completing the list examine it, and see how many men are in the list and how many women. Is it easy to think of male names or female names for each of the categories? Do some categories lend themselves to male rather than female, or *vice versa*? Why is this?

Communication across wider cultures is now possible. This has lead to a wider appreciation of differing attitudes to sexuality, increased awareness about sexual behaviours, and an understanding that such behaviours can be diverse. Defining what constitutes 'normal' sexual behviour is therefore loaded with ambiguities.

CONCLUSION

In the twentieth century there has been a 'freeing up' of conventions regarding sexual matters. There appears to be a progressive move towards a more tolerant and accepting society. Yet there is little doubt that there are some members of society who still believe in some of the historical perspective discussed in this chapter. Crudely, these could be divided into two opposing groups. One proposes that we develop our sexual feelings, attitudes, behaviour and love-making skills. While in opposition we are warned of the dangers of our sexuality, and that the strong emotions which are engendered should be kept under strict control. The messages about appropriate expression of sexuality come in various forms and strengths. This produces one common theme – sex is confusing (especially to the young). It is dirty and it is healthy, it is disgusting and it is beautiful, it is an expression of love and it is a physical act purely for the procreation of children. Whatever the answer to the complexities of the rights and wrongs of sexual expression, one factor remains constant – it is a powerful force. Society has attempted, with varying success, to control sexual expression. For the vast majority of people, sex is part of being alive. It is as natural and as important as eating and breathing. Being sexual is such a natural response that men and women have a sexual experience every 90 minutes while asleep. Men have erections, while women experience vaginal lubrication. Even young infants can have erections moments after birth (Masters and Johnson, 1966).

Freud points out that, psychologically, sexual expression is considerable, and that any suppression can have long-term effects on life. It has been suggested that sex within a relationship helps to bind the couple together. It is not purely a selfish act for pleasure, it helps to strengthen the importance of the family structure, and this in turn produces the efficacy around which the stability of a culture is built and maintained.

Sexuality should be a positive force in our lives; it warrants cultivation so that people of all ages can maximize its impact. This maximization should not be restricted to so-called 'normal heterosexual expression'. Sexuality has an enormous impact on people's lives; how we come to understand it and use it in a positive way is not easily answered. There are likely to be more questions than answers when looking at the subject of sexuality. For many people, discovering, discussing and applying sexuality in their lives will be a personal adventure. It is suggested that such an adventure leads to a greater understanding of ourselves and other people. The subject of sexuality is dynamic. By definition, then, the understanding of sexuality is a continuous, life-long process, and not an exact science. It is to this end that this book and the activities within it have been produced.

REFERENCES

Chesney, K. (1970) The Victorian underworld, in Hyam (1991) *Empire and Sexuality: The British Experience*, Manchester University Press.

Ellis, H. (1933) *Psychology of Sex*, Heinemann, London.

Feucht, O.E. (1961) (ed.) *Sex and the Church*, Mo Concordia, St Louis.

Forster, E.M. (1987) *Maurice*, Penguin Books, Harmondsworth, p. 196.

Foucault, M. (1979) *The History of Sexuality, Vol. 1.: An introduction*, translated by Hurley, R. Allen Lane, London.

Francome, C. (1979) More teenage sex. *Breaking Chains*. 11:7.

Freud, S. (1905) In *Sigmund Freud On Sexuality* (1991) (eds A. Richards and A. Dickson), Penguin Books, Harmondsworth.

Gay, P. (1986) The bourgeois experience. II: the tender passion, in Hyam (1991) *Empire and Sexuality: The British Experience*, Manchester University Press.

Godow, A.G. (1982) *Human Sexuality*, C.V. Mosby, St Louis.

Humphries, S. (1988) *A Secret World of Sex. Forbidden Fruit. The British Experience 1900–1950*, Sidgwick & Jackson, London.

Hyam, R. (1991) *Empire and Sexuality: The British Experience*, Manchester University Press.

Independent (1991) Sex education should start at five, say MPs, 7 November, p. 7.

Johnson, A.M., Wadsworth, J., Wellings, K. *et al.* (1992) Sexual lifestyles and HIV risk. *Nature*, **360**, 410–12.

Kinsey, A.C., Pomeroy, W.B. and Martin, C.E. (1948) *Sexual Behaviour in the Human Male*, W.B. Saunders, Philadelphia.

Kinsey, A.C., Pomeroy, W.B., Martin, C.E. *et al.* (1953) *Sexual Behaviour in the Human Female*, W.B. Saunders, Philadelphia.

Malinowski, B. (1963) *Sex, Culture and Myth*, Rupert Hart-Davis, London.

Masters, W.H. and Johnson, V.E. (1966) *Human Sexual Response*, Little, Brown, Boston.

Mead, M. (1964) *Sex and Temperament in Three Societies*, Routledge & Kegan Paul, London.

Padgug, R.A. (1979) Sexual matters: on conceptualizing sexuality in history. *Radical History Review*, No. 20. Spring/Summer. Special issue on *Sexuality in History*.

Tannahill, R. (1980) *Sex History*, Hamish Hamilton, London.

Weeks, J. (1989) *Sexuality*, Routledge, London.

CHAPTER 2

Definitions of sexuality

Sexuality means ... getting all dressed up and have men looking at me throughout the evening.

(First-year student nurse)

LEARNING OBJECTIVES

After reading this chapter you should be able to:

1. offer some definitions of sexuality;
2. understand that sexuality can be seen from different perspectives;
3. observe that various definitions offer different view points on sexuality.

Throughout this chapter there are a number of activities which are designed to help in your understanding of the subject under discussion. Notes for facilitators are provided where applicable so that discussion, if required, can take place within a group setting.

WHERE TO START?

The purpose of this chapter is to provide a literary vantage point from which to view the whole subject of sexuality. Hopefully, this will enable the reader to see some of the main themes and theories in the development of what is becoming a very complex topic. Indeed, the many facets of sexuality make the writing of its history somewhat troublesome (Freedman and D'Emilio, 1990). Just because we call it sexuality today does not mean that it has always been known by this term. This then presents us with a problem – how do we recount the history of sexuality when in the past it may have been known by other terms, or made up of different concepts? Of course, we have the work of famous writers such as Foucault (1979), Freud (1953) and Kinsey (1953), with the now famous *Kinsey*

Institute Report on Sex. Unfortunately, the four-volume work of Foucault on the history of sexuality makes for very complicated reading and, as such, offers little help to the casual reader. The remaining authors' work (Freud and Kinsey), although important, are lengthy and offer considerable debate on various ideas, findings from research, theories and concepts. Again, the enormity of this work is off-putting to the reader who just wants a simple explanation. The purpose of this chapter, and to some extent this book, is to open up these elaborate complexities so that the information becomes 'user friendly'. The prime aim is to present material which is understandable, usable and applicable to assist the nurse in caring for her patients. To assist in the perception and comprehension of sexuality, it may be helpful to consider the following analogy.

Imagine you are about to climb a mountain. Before you start you will probably have some preconceived ideas about what it will be like to climb, and the possible route you will take. So you walk around the mountain looking for a suitable path to start from. Yet as you walk around you notice that the mountain changes in the way it looks, so no matter which path you eventually use to climb, you will never be able to appreciate the whole mountain. To appreciate the mountain more fully you will have to climb it more than once, and from different routes. However, if you were to make the mountain your life's work and climb it from every possible angle, you would start (and only start) to appreciate the mountain as a whole. The same could be said about the concept of sexuality. As a concept it can be viewed and discussed from a range of angles or vantage points. It is the purpose of this book to take a predetermined path in our exploration of sexuality. This chapter will set up a 'base camp' so that the reader will have some appreciation of the complexities involved; in other words, the size, structure and difficulty of the mountain. Hopefully, this will lead to a clearer grasp of the possible origins of sexuality. The reader should bear in mind that, like mountain climbing, ours is not the only path.

First, we have to have some clear idea about the subject under discussion; in other words, we need a definition so that 'base camp' can be established and named. Before setting forth, it may be helpful to try the following activities:

Activity 1: Definitions

Using a piece of paper finish the following sentence: Sexuality means . . .

After you have completed the sentence, keep it on one side until the end of this chapter.

Activity 2: Definitions

A group of students are asked to complete the following sentence:
Sexuality means . . .

Facilitator's notes (time allowance 1.5 hours):

*Once each student has completed the sentence they should then join
with another student, sharing what they each have written. The students
either adopt what they consider to be the better of the two, or amalgamate
to produce a joint answer.*

*After two students have made a decision they then join another two
students (making four). They then decide to adopt one of the answers,
or attempt an amalgamation of all four answers.*

*After discussion, the facilitator asks each group of four to present their
answer. It is important to ask how the group arrived at the answer.
Also what was left out, and why. Can commonly occurring themes
be identified from what the students are saying? Are there various
concepts emerging? or do the responses pertain to the 'sex' side of
sexuality? It may be important to display the responses and see if
categorization can take place. For example; physical, psychological,
emotional, etc.*

DEFINITIONS

The Bible

The Bible is perhaps one of the first recorded discussions about sex
and sexuality. Throughout the *Old Testament* and *New Testament* there
are accounts on how people should behave when considering sexual
matters. Much of what is written tends to direct and guide people
in respect of their sexual feelings and actions. For example, *Leviticus*,
Chapter 18, verses six to 21, describes how improper incestuous relationships are:

> *None of you shall approach to any that is near of kin to him, to uncover
> their nakedness: I am the Lord. The nakedness of thy father, or the
> nakedness of thy mother, shalt thou not uncover (6–7).*

Further on in *Leviticus*, mention is made concerning homosexuality and bestiality:

Thou shall not lie with mankind, as with womankind: it is abomination. Neither shalt thou lie with any beast to defile thyself therewith: neither shall any woman stand before a beast to lie down thereto: it is confusion (22–4).

In *First Corinthians*, Chapter 6, verse nine, warning is given that those who are fornicators, idolaters, nor adulterers, nor effeminate, nor abusers of themselves with mankind shall inherit the Kingdom of God. These are strong words indeed for those who hold a strong belief and who cherish the words of *The Bible*. They serve to remind us of the fact that many people today still live their lives by the words in *The Bible*. Early forms of sex education used (literally) the teachings of *The Bible* in instructing young people in what was appropriate and inappropriate behaviour. Definitions of sexuality will be narrow for such people, and will revolve around do's and dont's, with dire consequences should desecrations occur.

World Health Organisation

In February 1974 the World Health Organisation (WHO) called a meeting of a group of health care professionals to discuss the concept of sexuality and the services directed towards sexual health. The concluding report of this meeting (WHO, 1975) gave the following definition of sexuality:

Sexual health is the integration of the somatic, emotional, intellectual and social aspects of sexual being, in ways that are positively enriching and that enhance personality, communication and love (p. 6).

You can be forgiven if, on first reading this definition, it is not clear what is being said. This is often the problem with definitions; they tend to be written by people who are immersed in the topic area, and as a consequence contain long-winded, complicated explanations which serve only to confuse rather than clarify the issue. So what does the WHO definition mean? It can be seen that sexuality is made up of a collection of other concepts – somatic, which means of the body or physical; emotional, meaning feelings affecting the psychology of the person; intellectual, implying cognitive understanding; and social, suggesting interaction with others.

The end result of having these components in harmony would 'enhance personality, communication and love'. This sounds a very laudable state of affairs, and one surely well worth striving for.

However, given that the subject of sexuality or sexual health receives little attention within the curriculum, let alone in the practice situation, do nurses have the insight and necessary skills to help patients achieve such a state?

The WHO report goes on to point out that while sexual health over the past few years has received little or no attention, its importance to the well-being and health of individuals is becoming increasingly essential. One only needs to consider the problems engendered by HIV and AIDS to see how true this is. Sadly, the curriculum in both medical and nursing schools still does not reflect the importance of sexuality as a subject (Webb and Askham, 1987).

The 'softer' side of being human

Hogan (1980) suggests sexuality is 'much more than the sex act; it is the quality of being human, all that we are as men and women, encompassing the most intimate feelings and deepest longings of the heart to find meaningful relationships'. This definition directs our attention to what may be called the 'softer' side of being human: intimate feelings and longings of the heart. Such sentiments conjure up images of romance (Mills and Boon stuff), falling in love, marriage and having a family. This 'non-sex act' is supported by other writers (see Savage, 1987). Stuart and Sundeen (1979) have a more all-encompassing explanation of sexuality. They say:

Sexuality is an integral part of the whole person. Human beings are sexual in every way, all the time. To a large extent human sexuality determines who we are. It is an integral factor in the uniqueness of every person. (p. 2).

This is an extremely broad view of things, the purpose of which leaves us with the notion that sexuality is an important complex factor present in us all. In essence, it generates more questions than answers. This global perspective is also supported by Lion (1982), who states that 'sexuality is all that being human is, it runs through every facet of our life from birth through to death'. Sexuality is part of being human, reflected in our character and personality, in how we see the world, and how we think the world should see us. Such a view invites us to consider our self-concept and self-esteem. Self-concept is a useful notion in aiding our understanding because it allows consideration of the physical, emotional and social domains of an individual. Those people with a good self-concept respect themselves and consider themselves to be worthwhile people. This, of course, does not mean that they are better than others, they just have a stronger identity of self. The alternative to this is low self-concept where the person does not value their own worth. They have a negative perspective which, depending on its strength, could lead to self-rejection. This view of sexuality asks us to examine our self-concept and the relationships we have (or do not have) with the wider society. Such a definition of sexuality is a very personal one and comes out of people's personality, how we think we project ourselves to others, and what others think of us.

A natural phenomenon

Sexuality could also be viewed as a natural phenomenon, in other words, it is with us from the day we are born – an innate almost natural force or inclination. There is some genetic research to support the fact that man is not controlled by his loins, but rather it is the result of the DNA in his chromosomes that makes him behave in a particular way (Wilson, 1975). Work which looks at the sexual activity of primates and prehistoric man suggests that there was a swing between monogamy and polygamy, a swing which was related directly to the weather and living conditions of the time. Climatic conditions in those very early days would most certainly affect survival. It is the central struggle for life, the act of survival and reproduction that has been passed down (in our genes) from our ancestors.

If this is true then it would appear that our acts of procreation are driven not by a desire for love, but by the determination of our genes to propagate themselves. This has been the thinking behind most of the prominent and eminent writers on sexuality (see Freud and Kinsey). They suggest that this instinctive, even 'animal' type of human behaviour is present no matter what forces are about to control it. This overpowering urge is evident through our sexual activity; activity which falls either within socially acceptable behaviour, or behaviour which is seen as perverse. The amount or degree of such behaviour, whether perverse or normal, varies from culture to culture, and is also dependent on the particular circumstances in which we find ourselves. The instinctive theory is not supported by later writers (Gagnon and Simon, 1973), who believe that sexuality is a consequence of social interactions.

Sexuality is learned by picking up cues from those around us, from our social environment and the culture we live in. Such a notion may help our understanding of different, or what some may call deviant, types of sexual behaviour or inclination being a consequence of one's environment. This idea could go some way towards explaining why those people who were sexually abused as children then go on to sexually abuse their own children. The whole area of child abuse is complex and one which is beyond the scope of this book. Those requiring further information should see Carver (1980) and Porter (1987).

Another definition of sexuality can be derived from the purely biological function. Or as Hohmann (1972) succinctly describes it:

A biological act that involves the build-up of both autonomic nervous system and striated muscle activity that culminates in orgasm. It is a biological force that is necessary for the procreation of the human race (p. 50).

What Hohmann is saying is that, whether we like it or not, part of our hormones and genetic make-up affects our sexuality. We should make the distinction here that sex and sexuality are not one and the same thing. Sex relates more to the physiological act and the biological state. Sexuality is a broader term which includes the biological as well as the cultural, social, psychological and moral components of our sexual behaviour.

A physiological need

The final definition of sexuality comes from the writings of Maslow (1954) and his theory of human motivation, which is derived from needs in relation to health, and has sex as one of the basic physiological needs. Other basic needs are: oxygen, food and water, elimination, rest, activity and shelter. These he calls the basic survival needs.

However, the need for sexual activity seems out of place in such a list, as it is not absolutely necessary for individual survival; but it is essential if the species is to survive. The higher order needs Maslow mentions, namely, security, love, belonging, esteem and, finally, self-actualization, have significant implications when considering the concept of sexuality. The term self-actualization could be described as being at one with yourself and others, a sort of fusion of all that is important to you. It is important to ask yourself whether this is ever possible; it could be just an ideal state which on occasions we reach at points in our lives. Each of these superior needs has a seam of sexuality running through it, and as such joins each of these higher needs together. In order to self-actualize you have to have some sort of sexual identity and cohesiveness with all of the needs Maslow describes. For most of us this will mean spending a large proportion of our lives attempting to balance these needs with what is available; our ability to do this will affect how happy and contented we are with our lives.

Whichever of the above definitions is chosen to understand the image of sexuality, it is of paramount importance to remember that sexuality is what being human is, it is not an exact science. It is the expression of one or more, usually two, individuals who merge together with symbolic and physical feelings of love and respect for each other.

Such an expression is bound up in desire and pleasure, of which there should be a mutuality about the relationship between others as well as the self.

So what do all these definitions give us?

Well, with each of these definitions there seems to be one common denominator – that the concept of sexuality is multifarious. It is made up of a collection of physical, psychological and social elements; it is about how we are as individuals, how we react with each other, and the society we live in; what comfort we derive from each, and the importance we attach to belonging, being loved and loving. In an effort to understand the above definitions, try the following activities, 3 and 4.

Activity 3: A bit of what you fancy does you good

Stop for a moment and think about the relationships you have had with girlfriends/boyfriends, or consider the relationship you are in at the moment. Try and answer the following questions:

1. What was the first thing that attracted you to the other person?
2 When you look at people of the opposite sex what are the first things you look for?
3. What do you think women find attractive about other women?
4. What do you think men find attractive about other men?

Facilitator's notes (time allowance 45 minutes):

Ask group members to sit in a large circle, so that everybody can be seen and heard. The facilitator then explains the activity, and allows for those who do not wish to take part to say 'pass'. The facilitator invites each person in turn to respond to each of the four questions.

A discussion follows in which the facilitator attempts to tie up themes, and discovers where people have gathered their views and opinions from.

Activity 4: What I find attractive about you is . . .

Ask the group to sit in a large circle, so everybody can be seen and heard. The facilitator then explains the activity, and allows for those who do not wish to take part to say 'pass'.

The facilitator turns to the person on the right and says, 'What a man would find attractive about you is ... ' (and finishes the sentence). It is important that the gender does not change, even as in this instance it is said to another man. This person then turns to the next person and repeats the procedure. This process is continued until all the group members have taken a turn. The process can be repeated by using the opposite gender.

Facilitator's notes (time allowance 40 minutes):

It is important in this activity that people are not pressured into taking part.

The facilitator then asks, 'What did that feel like?' or, 'What did you discover?'

During the ensuing discussion it might be helpful to ask the students to identify where they think the feelings they had are generated.

A RESEARCH PROJECT

Like any textbook, these definitions are fine and very helpful when one has to write a project or essay on sexuality. Such things usually start with definitions. But what would be interesting to find out is, what does the concept of sexuality mean to the average student nurse or qualified nurse working on the ward? How do they view the concept of sexuality? To find the answer to these questions we conducted a small-scale research project with first-, second- and third-year student nurses and qualified staff. They were asked to complete the sentence which read: 'Sexuality means ... ' This 'snap-shot' of people's understanding produced the following range of responses.

First-year student nurses

Sexuality means ...

1. 'Attracting the opposite sex, even if you haven't gone out to do so.'
2. 'A person's personal feelings towards others.'
3. 'The way males and females express themselves in manner, appearance, sexual preferences and opinions.'
4. 'A way in which a person portrays their own sexuality by the way they look, dress, maintain their personal appearance and by what role they play in society.'

5. 'How somebody expresses themselves to others by using their charms, body language, looks and body.'
6. 'Being able to be yourself.'
7. 'Being able to be feminine but equal in a relationship.'
8. 'Being a women, mother and a wife but *also* an individual.'
9. 'The way in which others perceive you or the way you would like to be perceived as a person.'

These short responses offer some insight into what first-year students are thinking, and their attitudes towards sexuality. An analysis of the answers show they range from attraction (1), feelings (2), appearance (3 and 4), physical expression (3 and 5), gender identity (4, 7 and 8), the concept of self (6) and, finally, role identity (4 and 8). It would appear that for a predominantly young group of people, they have a broad understanding of the components involved in sexuality. Such knowledge, possibly, has something to do with how the subject matter is treated by today's society and the media. This subject will be returned to later in this chapter when the treatment of sexuality through history is considered.

Third-year student nurses

Sexuality means . . .

1. 'Sexuality is a means of distinguishing oneself or others via means of personality, appearance, experience, and incorporating it into society of the present.'
2. 'A physical, spiritual, emotional state of being or awareness.'
3. 'The way you perceive yourself, in your own right, as a whole which is often due to upbringing and past experiences.'
4. 'An individual's expression of his or her masculinity or femininity, including their role as mother, daughter, sister, etc.'
5. 'The way in which we present ourselves in appearance, behaviour, speech and attitudes, and beliefs.'
6. 'An individual seen as mind, body and soul.'
7. 'An interpretation of how a person portrays him or herself to the outside world. I understand that sexuality is very personal.'
8. 'What I am, to myself not to others, my individuality.'

An analysis of these answers shows definitions ranging from – appearance (1 and 5), expression to self and outside world (7 and 8), gender and role identity (4), upbringing and past experiences (3), physical, emotional, spiritual (2 and 6). Again, like the first-year students, these third-year students understand sexuality to be a complex phenomenon made up of various aspects. Yet the depth of the response shows little movement from the statements made by the first-year students, which is surprising given the extent of experience the students will have had at this point in their training. The possible reason for this could be related to the lack of time or opportunity given for discussion and teaching within the curriculum. Attention is directed towards discussing this view in Chapter 9, on the teaching of sexuality.

Qualified nurses

Sexuality means . . .

1. 'How a person perceives oneself sexually to self and others. How they see their body image.'
2. 'The ability of males and females to express themselves within their own gender and to express their sexual needs and dress to each other.'
3. 'How one perceives oneself and the perception others have of you.'
4. 'The expression of an individual's gender via a variety of communication methods.'
5. 'How people express their sexual orientation and feelings about the subject.'
6. 'How a person functions sexually, but it is a complex factor. It is reflected in how a person presents him/herself to the world, their self-esteem and self-confidence.'
7. 'How I feel/what I do to make me feel the way I do/how I interpret all the above and more.'
8. 'The portrayal of a person as a whole. Their looks, gestures, language, facial expression and dress. Sexuality is not simply sex.'

An analysis of these responses shows the areas covered as: the concept of self (1, 3 and 6), gender and role identity (2 and 4), feelings (5 and 7), and various methods of communication (4 and 8).

Like the responses of the first- and second-year students, a commonly occurring theme appears to be the complexity of the subject, the fact that it does not stand alone with a set of clearly defined boundaries. What this small piece of work tells us is, in fact, what the collective nature of the previous definitions has attempted to detail.

At this point it might be of value to return to activity 1, which was set at the start of this chapter (p. 27). Look at your response and compare it to the statements made above.

It should be borne in mind that the above small-scale research is by no means a representative piece of work. What it offers is some ideas. It might be interesting to repeat the procedure with similar or different groups of people or professionals to discover whether perceptions are the same.

The discussions above have covered a great deal of ground; before moving on it may be wise to consolidate the debate so far. This is done by presenting flow charts, which are structured in such a way that they expose the salient points of each of the definitions discussed previously. The chapter concludes with four activities which should personalize the understanding of sexuality and its many definitions. These activities can be carried out either individually or within a group setting.

FLOW CHARTS OF DEFINITIONS

Do's and dont's

(The Bible)

Directions on right and wrong behaviour
Importance of procreation not fornication
Incestuous relationships
Homosexuality
Bestiality
Consequences of improper actions

Systems view

(World Health Organisation)

Somatic
Emotional
Intellectual
Social

Global view

(Hogan)

'The softer side of sexuality'
Much more than the sexual act
It is about being human
Intimate feelings
Relationships

Personal view

(Lion)

Runs through all facets of life
The continuum of birth to death

Character
Personality
Perceptions of 'self' and world

Natural phenomenon view

(Freud)

Instinctive behaviour
Animal-like
Behaviour controlled by society
Perverse behaviour due to lack of control

Sociological view

(Gagnon and Simon)

Social interactions
Social environment/culture
Learned behaviour

Biological/physiological function view

(Hohmann)

Autonomic nerve and muscle activity
Hormones
Sexual act

Motivational or needs view

(Maslow)

Need for sexual activity
Security
Love
Belonging
Esteem
Self-actualization

Activity 5: Mental images

Part A. When you hear the word 'sexuality' what does it conjure up in your mind, what mental images do you see? Jot down your ideas on a piece of paper. Or can you attempt to draw images of them?

Part B. Once you have completed part A, ask yourself where your images come from.

Facilitator's note (time allowance 1 hour):

If this is done in a large group, each individual should first answer part A and B, and then share their answers with a small group of about six people. The group should then identify common and uncommon themes that are occurring in the answers. The group then reports back to a large group if necessary. The group facilitator should outline the major areas identified.

Activity 6: Read all about it

Pick up a magazine or newspaper and thumb through the pages. As you do so, make a note of how often you think the concept of sexuality is used. Those magazines that use a considerable amount of photographs and advertisements are best for this type of exercise. Try discussing your thoughts with others and see if they share your opinions or point of view. Ask yourself during the course of discussions how you think you have arrived at your particular viewpoint. Do others share your perception of things?

Facilitator's note (time allowance 1.5 hours):

The items identified from the media can be cut out and a group asked to form a collection or collage, which it then presents under a suggested heading. You might consider forming the presentation as if it were an exhibition of art with a theme and title to each picture. Students should then give a 'conducted tour' of their work, and offer explanations. Attempts should be made to discuss and discover how people perceive the images, and where their perceptions come from.

Activity 7: Stop me and buy one

Next time you watch television, note how often you consider the notion of sexuality is used. It may be interesting to consider advertisements only and how the notion of sexuality is used to sell a particular product. Some advertisement agencies use obvious sexuality while others use a more subtle, almost subliminal approach. See if you can identify which are which.

Facilitator's note (time allowance 1 hour):

To use this exercise for a large group, record a selection of advertisements, play each in turn to the group, and ask:

1. *Is this sexual?*
2. *How is it using sexuality?*
3. *How have you arrived at your opinions?*
4. *Does everybody share the same opinions?*

It may be helpful to jot down and display the major themes that emerge from the discussions.

Activity 8: Whose perception?

Please read the following short descriptions:

A. George is 36. He is a homosexual in a solid and loving relationship which has been going for the last 10 years. George and his partner have been faithful to each other. They both have good jobs, and have a wide circle of friends. Most of the time they keep themselves to themselves and are respected members of the community.

B. Joe is an attractive 19-year-old. He has a wide circle of friends with whom he usually goes out at least three times a week. Joe and his friends live life to the full even if this means getting a little boisterous when they have had a bit to drink. Joe has had a regular girlfriend since he was 16. However, at least once a month he has sex with a different girl.

C. Les is 40, married with two children. Les and his wife have a deep, loving relationship. For the last three years Les has been having frequent affairs, but he has never told his wife, nor does he intend to do so.

D. Victoria is 20. She is single but has a steady boyfriend of three years' standing; they are both saving up to get married. Although Victoria loves her boyfriend she has never 'gone all the way' when making love. She was brought up as a strict Catholic, and both her parents go to church regularly. Victoria stopped going to church as soon as she was able.

Now look at the following continuum:

Acceptable ——— ——— ——— ——— ——— Unacceptable
            1   2   3   4   5

Fill in the continuum by placing the letter of each of the descriptions where you think it should be. For example, if you consider 'A' to be acceptable behaviour then place the letter 'A' over the number 1. If you consider it to be unacceptable behaviour, then place the letter 'A' over number 5, and so on, until each of the four have been rated.

Facilitator's note (time allowance 1 hour):

The facilitator should invite answers to the following questions (this being done alone or in groups):

1. What reasons can you offer for placing them as you did?
2. Show this exercise to one of your parents and ask them to complete it. Compare your answers. If they differ, why do they differ?
3. Reverse the gender in each of the above, so that George becomes Georgina; Joe becomes Josephine; Les becomes Lesley; and Victoria becomes Vic. Construct another continuum. Does this make a difference in your ranking? If it does, why does it?

Once a particular group has identified where the men lie in the ranking, ask another group (who have ranked the women) to persuade the male group to change their mind, and accept their point of view.

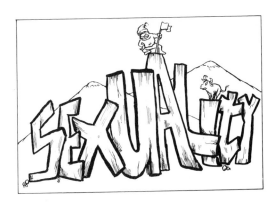

REFERENCES

Carver, V. (ed.) (1980) *Child Abuse: A Study Text*, The Open University Press, Milton Keynes.

Foucault, M. (1979) *The History of Sexuality, Volume 1: An Introduction* (translated by R. Hurley), Allen Lane, London.

Freedman, E.B. and D'Emilio, J. (1990) Problems encountered in writing the history of sexuality: sources, theory and interpretation. *The Journal of Sex Research*, **27**, 481–95.

Freud, S. (1953, reprinted 1991) 7. *On Sexuality. Three Essays on the Theory of Sexuality and Other Works*, Penguin Books, Harmondsworth.

Gagnon, J. and Simon, W. (1973) *Sexual Construct: The Social Sources of Human Sexuality*, Aldine Publishing, Chicago.

Hogan, R. (1980) *Human Sexuality. A Nursing Perspective*, Appleton-Century-Crofts, New York.

Hohmann, G.N. (1972) Considerations in management of psychosexual readjustment in the cord injured male. *Rehabilitation Psychology*, **19**, 50–58.

Kinsey, A.C., Pomeroy, W.B. and Martin, C.E. (1953) *Sexual Behaviour in the Human Female*, W.B. Saunders, Philadelphia.

Lion, E.M. (ed.) (1982) *Human Sexuality in the Nursing Process*, John Wiley, New York.

Maslow, A. (1954) *Motivation and Personality*, Harper & Row, New York.

Porter, R. (ed.) (1987) *Child Sexual Abuse Within the Family*, Ciba Foundation/Tavistock, London.

Savage, J. (1987) *Nursing Today. Nurses' Gender and Sexuality*, Heinemann Nursing, London.

Stuart, G.W. and Sundeen, S.J. (eds) (1979) *Principles and Practice of Psychiatric Nursing*, C.V. Mosby, St Louis.

Webb, C. and Askham, J. (1987) Nurses' knowledge and attitudes about sexuality in health care – a review of the literature. *Nurse Education Today*, **7**, 75–87.

Wilson, E.O. (1975) *Sociobiology: The New Synthesis*, Cambridge University Press, Cambridge, UK.

World Health Organisation (1975) *Education and Treatment in Human Sexuality: The Training of Health Professionals. Report of a WHO meeting*, WHO, Geneva.

CHAPTER 3

Sexuality and ethics

LEARNING OBJECTIVES

A brief general discussion of ethics and its relevance to nursing will be followed by its more specific application to sexuality. Implications will be discussed from the patient's as well as the nurse's point of view. After reading this chapter you should be able to:

1. have a general idea of ethics and its importance to nursing;
2. be able to discuss the main principles and issues regarding sexuality and nursing from:
   (i) the nurse's point of view;
   (ii) the patient's point of view.

WHAT IS ALL THIS ABOUT ETHICS?

Ethics is becoming an important part of nurse education, both at pre- and post-registration level. But what exactly does ethics mean and why should we know about it?

Ethics is about activities; it involves thinking about morality and deciding between right and wrong, between good and bad. Such decisions are obviously not made in a vacuum; we all have some basic ideas regarding what is good and what is bad.

Because ethics is essentially something you 'do', this chapter is structured around activities, which hopefully will enable you to get an idea of what ethical reasoning is all about.

Activity 1

Spend some time thinking about some essential values and principles that you hold, and which form the basis of your general view of life and the way you feel that you and others should act.

Discussion

When people are asked to do this activity there is often a remarkable consistency in their answers. Here are some:

- honesty, being truthful;
- freedom;
- respect for others;
- not hurting others;
- treating others as you want to be treated yourself;
- privacy.

Did you include any of these values in your list? It may be interesting to ask a few other people the same question and see what answers they come up with. You will probably find that there is quite a degree of overlap, although you may have some values which appear to be very much your own. Even if you and your friends produced different lists, the chances are that you will agree with each other's lists, or at least not disagree too much.

WHERE DO VALUES COME FROM?

We are all born into a particular environment, which includes our family, our culture and our society. As a consequence, our values are likely to reflect those of our environment. However, that is not to say that people who are born into the same environment necessarily end up having the same values. We all know that things are not that straightforward and that people from the same family may argue violently about things.

Also, society is changing continuously and we adapt to those changes all of the time. Particularly where sexuality is concerned, as we saw in Chapter 1, there have been many changes over time and no doubt there will be many more.

General values and principles very much reflect common values held by most people. However, the way people **use** these values and principles in everyday life may differ. Different people may give different weightings to things depending on their own theoretical stance, cultural or religious or family background, or depending on the specific situation.

RELEVANCE TO HEALTH CARE

It could be said that all work for health is a moral endeavour. This is because whatever position you hold, whatever work you do, it involves the well-being of others. The work that you do affects others, whether directly or indirectly. It is likely that what you do from day to day is affected by values, which you have chosen from alternatives. If you are a student nurse, for example, your work may be inspired by a value of 'doing good', or by 'health' itself. Perhaps you value health so highly that you wish to help people to preserve or regain it wherever possible.

PRINCIPLES

In health care it is generally agreed that the following principles apply, although this list is by no means exhaustive (Seedhouse, 1988):

- autonomy;
- beneficence (doing good);
- non-maleficence (not causing harm);
- truth telling;
- respect for people;
- promise keeping.

This list of basic, generally agreed principles is very similar to the list people usually come up with. They are useful when you are faced with having to make an ethical decision. For example, a patient may ask to be told her diagnosis only for you to find out that she has not been told the truth. A number of principles are involved here. Obviously the principle of 'truth telling' has not been abided by, and the principle of non-maleficence may also be involved.

Quite likely not telling the truth has been done with the best of intentions, according to the principle of 'non-maleficence'. It might have been thought that the patient would get so upset if she heard the truth that it would do her harm. In order to decide what to do you have to reason things out, to balance the good and the harm. You may well think that a greater harm will come to the patient if she finds out later that she has been lied to.

It is also useful to look at the consequences of particular actions (consequences for all concerned). In the above example you may think that the consequences of not telling the truth may be a lack of trust between the patient and the people caring for her. This way of ethical decision making is called 'consequentialism' and has two main components: (1) 'what is of value', and, having decided what is of value, that (2) 'more of it is better than less'.

So, from a consequentialist viewpoint it is better to carry out 200 hip operations than one heart operation, as the choice is between relieving suffering for 200 people rather than just one person. In health care, decisions are often made from a consequentialist point of view.

DO WE SEE IT AS OUR BUSINESS?

Scenario

A staff nurse was overheard saying, 'If I come in with an ingrowing toenail I don't want someone asking me about my sexuality. The type of shoes I wear has nothing to do with it.'

Her colleague answered, 'Yes they have, they are part of how you express your sexuality.'

First nurse: 'OK, but I don't want to be asked about it.'

Second nurse: 'Yes, but of course there may be a direct link between your ingrowing toenail and the fact that you wear five-inch heels.'

First nurse: 'Leave my heels alone. I don't feel right without them.'

Second nurse: 'There you are, then, that proves my point.'

Although we live in an overtly sexual society and are constantly bombarded with sexual images via the media, we do not talk easily about our own sexuality. Indeed, we may feel, as the nurse in the above conversation, that to be questioned about our sexuality is an invasion of our privacy.

If that is how we feel about our own sexuality, how do we feel about including sexuality in our overall nursing care? What exactly is it all about?

WHAT DO NURSES REALLY THINK?

It needs only a fairly cursory scrutiny of the nursing literature to realize that the idea of holistic care, involving physical, psychosocial and spiritual care appears to be well established within nursing. Most nursing models and theories are based on the holistic idea. The Roper model, for example, which is used widely within British health care, specifically includes 'expressing sexuality' as one of the activities of living (Roper, Logan and Tierney, 1980). And, as is the case with all the other activities of living such as breathing, sleeping or mobility, patients have to be assessed on it.

But, writing about it is one thing, doing it is another. Do nurses agree with the inclusion of sexuality in holistic care? And, if they agree that it should be part of nursing care, do they actually do it and, if so, how?

Facts

We asked 61 nurses (16 second-year students and 45 qualified people) to complete the following sentence:

'When discussing the activity of sexuality the other day, one nurse turned to me and said, it is none of our business anyway. I think . . . '

The answers given fell into four categories:

1. 'Yes, it is our business as part of holistic care.'
2. 'Yes, it is our business as illness can affect sexuality.'
3. 'It depends.'
4. 'No, it is none of our business.'

Yes, it is our business as part of holistic care

This was the largest group, numbering 29 (14 students, 15 qualified). Typical statements included the following.

- 'I think it is the nurse's business as nursing staff can assess how the patient expresses sexuality and what is usually normal for the patient' (qualified nurse).
- 'I think sexuality is our business as it is what many of us portray to the outside world and is vitally important. It does not necessarily mean a deep discussion regarding sexual behaviour or idiosyncrasies, perversions, etc' (qualified nurse).
- 'I think we need to know about the patient's ways of expressing sexuality in order to care for them holistically' (student).
- 'I think that to enable us to gain an overall view of a patient's preferred way of life, we need to obtain knowledge on their sexuality as part of their life and so enabling holistic care to be given' (student).

Yes it is our business – specific

Fourteen qualified nurses gave specific examples of how illness can affect sexuality and how nurses can help. Examples included the following.

- 'It is part of rehabilitation information that we give to patients post-infarct.'
- 'It can be important if a lady has undergone a mastectomy and has an altered body image.'
- 'If the patient was going for surgery, for example, positioning of the scar may be possible or in the case of mutilating surgery, it will alter their self-image. The same may apply following a myocardial infarction where the person may believe they are only half the person they were.'

It depends

Twelve qualified nurses thought that it depends on the patient, the condition or the situation. Examples included the following.

- 'If the circumstances are relevant then it is our business.'
- 'It is a personal issue but it may be relevant to her care, so you'd have to be careful how you ask about her sexuality.'

No, it is none of our business

Six people (almost 10%) fell into this category (four qualified, two students). Answers included statements such as the following.

- 'I think that nurse is correct. Each person's business is their own personal choice' (qualified).
- 'I agree with her! Unless the patient offers this kind of information, I don't think we should pursue it' (qualified).
- 'Each to their own. Who are we to judge others about their sexual practices?' (student).

Thus approximately two-thirds of our 'snap-shot sample' did see the activity of expressing sexuality as having a part in nursing care, although only a minority gave concrete examples. Most people, especially students, seemed to have only a vague idea as to what is involved, whereas almost one-tenth of the nurses thought that sexuality 'is none of our business'.

Approximately one-fifth qualified their answers by saying something like, 'It depends on the patient's problems as to whether it is relevant or not', which suggests that some nurses assess the situation and then decide whether or not to include 'expressing sexuality' in their overall care of a particular patient.

Activity 2

'It depends on the patient's problem whether the activity of sexuality is relevant or not.'

Consider the above statement for a few moments. What are the implications?

Discussion

There are a number of issues here. First, although 'expressing sexuality' is supposed to be one of the activities of living, it is not always regarded as relevant. It is not clear what the criteria are for deciding whether or not it is relevant, although 'the patient's condition' may be one factor. Second, nurses imply that they assess people in order to decide on the relevance.

This argument may be put more formally as follows:

- Sexuality may or not be relevant;
- There are criteria for deciding this relevance;
- Therefore nurses need to (1) know these criteria; (2) have the skills to assess people on these criteria.

Chapters 4 and 5 will discuss in more detail all the issues related to assessment. However, it is interesting and slightly worrying that, perhaps because they are not totally comfortable with an issue, nurses redefine their position without realizing that they have done so.

In other words, on the one hand they say 'Yes, sexuality is very much a part of our everyday lives and therefore part of overall holistic nursing care', whereas on the other hand they say, 'Hang on a minute, sexuality is not always relevant; it all depends. We have to assess each situation on its merits.' The two positions appear to be contradictory; either the one is true and the other false, or *vice versa*. We have to make up our minds in order to be clear about what we should be doing.

WHAT DO NURSES ACTUALLY DO?

If we assume that most nurses agree that sexuality should be included in overall nursing care, how is it done? To think it is a good idea is one thing, to actually do it is another.

Activity 3

Go to a clinical area, preferably the one where you are working at present, and select 10 patients' records at random. Have a look at the 'expressing sexuality' section of the nursing assessment. What is written down? Are problems identified? Is relevance decided upon, and if so, according to what criteria?

Discussion

If your experience is the same as ours, you will probably be feeling rather disappointed.

Assessment is the first stage of nursing care from which all else follows. We therefore decided to find out what nurses actually do when they assess a patient on the activity of expressing sexuality.

We asked 32 qualified nurses to complete the following sentence: 'When assessing a patient on the activity of sexuality I usually ...'

Answers fell into two categories:

1. Comments on appearance and/or marital status.
2. Assessment of whether the illness or surgery may affect the activity.

One person said that she would avoid this subject, another commented that she used the holistic approach and therefore did not assess using activities of living.

Comments on appearance and/or marital status

Two-thirds (21) of the answers fell into this category. Typical comments included the following.

*   'Recap their marital status from admission slip and look at their overall appearance, for example, hair, clothes, etc.'
*   'Ask whether patient is married, engaged or has a partner. Look at patient's overall appearance – whether or not he/she is well groomed, wears make-up, etc.'
*   'I usually observe the patient for the wearing of, for example, make-up, jewellery, whether they are well dressed, their hair looked after or if a man is well-shaven or has a beard.'

Assess whether the illness/surgery may affect the activity

Nine people fell into this category. The answers included statements such as the following.

*   'If I thought it was relevant, for example, if a lady was in for a mastectomy or a disfiguring operation, or a disease that caused sexual dysfunction.'
*   'I am acutely aware of body image and I will discuss this if, for example, surgery is planned regarding stoma, mastectomy or any ablative surgery.'
*   'It should be the nurse's role to counsel patients on how the illness or treatment might affect the patient's body image, for example, skin complaints, scarring, etc.'

From these answers it is clear that the majority of people comment on the patient's appearance and find out whether they have a partner, but that less than one-third consider how the activity of sexuality may be affected by the current physical problem or treatment.

So it appears that at times there is a gap between what we say and what we do. There are three possible explanations for this discrepancy:

1. The nurse in the conversation at the beginning of this chapter was right after all; perhaps nurses do feel deep down that it is not really any of their business.
2. Nurses have a very superficial idea of holistic care in general and the activity of sexuality in particular.
3. Nurses realize their shortcomings but do not know how to overcome them, as they have not really been prepared adequately.

A further scrutiny of the answers given above by the nurses indicates that the second and third explanations may be the case. The two types of explanation are related; if a nurse has not really learned how to assess a patient holistically it may follow that she has only a superficial idea of holistic care.

HOLISTIC CARE

Sometimes the nursing and medical professions are accused of paternalism, of thinking they know what is best for a patient, rather than the patient herself. A well-known consequence of paternalism is not giving a patient accurate information about the diagnosis, sometimes even to the extent of not telling a patient that she is terminally ill, for example.

Some people might like to argue that to assess a patient holistically is an example of that paternalism. If a patient comes in for a particular problem, such as a stomach complaint, for example, she may not realize that nurses and doctors are going to look further than the immediately obvious problem. Patients may have a 'let's get it fixed' approach to whatever is the matter with them, and may not realize that the presenting problem may be related to other, not immediately obvious, factors.

The woman with the stomach complaint, for example, may just want it diagnosed accurately and then given the appropriate treatment, whether that involves surgery or drugs or both. She may not necessarily appreciate or understand the importance of investigations into her diet, lifestyle or stress levels. Even if she does understand the importance, she may not necessarily like it, and may resent intrusions into what she may regard as her private life.

Also, if we carry out a holistic assessment, we may discover problems unrelated to the original presenting problem yet which, in our professional opinion, need to be looked into.

Activity 4

Find a few colleagues and discuss the following questions:

'Do you think we should look further than the presenting problem?'

'Do we have a right to carry out a holistic assessment without the patient realizing what we are doing?'

Discussion

To the first question you may have answered that, as we have a duty to give the best possible care, we must investigate a problem adequately, even if the investigation goes further than the patient expects. If we did not do this, we might overlook important information and the patient could suffer as a result. So, not to investigate a problem properly could be regarded as negligence. Rights imply duties, in other words, if one person has a right, someone else has a duty to provide it. In this case, the patient has a right to adequate care, therefore we have a duty to provide it.

What about the second question; is it different from the first? If we say that a patient has a right to the best possible care, then it could be argued that we have a duty to carry out a holistic assessment. That is because only a holistic assessment is likely to bring to light all the problems a patient may have, and which we can do something about. And as we have a duty to care, we must carry out the assessment in order to find out what we can do.

Activity 5

'Only a holistic assessment is likely to reveal all the problems a patient may have. Therefore, as we have a duty to care, we have a duty to carry out a holistic assessment.'

Think about the above argument. Do you agree with it? Please give reasons for your answer.

Discussion

This is very difficult, and you may have a gut feeling that you simply always want to do whatever is best for the patient. Surely that must involve a holistic assessment. Yes, you are probably right. But what we must also do is talk to people, inform them of what it is we are planning to do, explain our reasons and ask their permission. Traditionally we have been very bad at keeping patients informed about what it is we actually do for them and why. If, to go back to the example at the beginning of this chapter, someone comes in for an ingrowing toenail and is then asked all sorts of questions about breathing, bowel habits and sexuality, they are entitled first of all to know why these questions are asked and, second, they have the right not to answer.

In other words, they are entitled to give their 'informed consent'. The principle of informed consent does not just apply to giving a surgeon permission to carry out a particular operation. It involves absolutely everything. Really, nurses should never do anything to a patient unless they have agreed to it; not to do so is, technically speaking, assault. It is not necessary to ask a patient to sign a consent form every time a nurse takes her blood pressure – the fact that she holds out her arm for the nurse to carry on is enough, and implies that she agreed with what the nurse is going to do.

What is important is to talk to people and to give them adequate information; to question a patient on bowel habits or sexuality without an explanation and without getting their permission to do so is an invasion of privacy and violates the idea of informed consent.

Activity 6

Read again through the above discussion and look back at the ethical principles outlined at the beginning of this chapter. Which principle/s would you say is/are relevant to informed consent?

Discussion

The main principle relevant to informed consent is that of autonomy. We are all autonomous human beings and as such have the right to decide what to do and how to live our lives. Consequently, we have the right to decide whether we want a particular investigation or treatment. Logically, the right to informed consent implies the right to informed non-consent, the right to say no.

WHAT DO PATIENTS WANT?

Having investigated some of the issues surrounding assessing patients on the activity of sexuality in particular and holistic assessment in general, it is time to turn things around and look at it from the patient's point of view.

We know, on the whole, how we feel and what our views are, but what is it that patients want and expect?

Scenario

Imagine you are lying in a hospital bed waiting to be examined by the doctor. You have been admitted and are obviously a little anxious. A young nurse comes up to you and says, 'Do you mind if I ask you a few questions? It is part of our assessment and will help us to know how best to look after you.'

She then asks you a range of questions, most of which appear to be about bodily functions. You are not at all sure why she wants to know all this as it does not seem very relevant to your actual problem. You answer politely. After all, they know what they are doing and it is actually quite nice to have an interest shown in you. It also helps to pass the time. And then she asks, 'What about your sexuality, any problems?'

How would you react? Surprised? Shocked? Angry? Pleased?

Conversation

The above example was discussed with a group of women, none of whom were nurses. Their reaction was one of surprise. Why on earth would the nurse ask that, surely it was none of her business? Were they trying to find out if there was a risk of HIV?

The above example was obviously a bit crude; hopefully nobody would come out with the question just like that. However, it made this author think whether or not patients really want what we think they want. Do they know they are being assessed holistically and, if so, do they agree with it?

The group had all been in hospital at some stage in their lives, and all had also had experience of relatives and friends in hospital. The following is a resumé of the discussion that took place.

First, they were asked, 'What is your impression of nurses? What is it they do?' Their answers included statements such as, 'They look after your physical needs', and, 'The good ones can give you the information you require; it is easier as they are closer to you than the doctors.'

Others, however, said that in their experience the qualified nurses were far too busy to spend much time with the patients, and that it was actually the nursing auxiliaries who were the most helpful.

They were then asked, 'What would you like nurses to do?'

Most said that they would like a more free contact with the qualified nurses so that they could ask questions as and when they occurred. Particular examples were information regarding time needed off work, explanations of what kind of operation had actually been done, and advice on lifestyle or diet.

One woman said, 'The good ones treat you as if you have a mind as well as a body. But to others it is just routine, you are just another person having a hysterectomy, or a breast lump removed.'

It was then explained that nures were now expected to assess people holistically and to deliver holistic care. 'But how can you expect that from a 21-year-old?' was one reaction. 'How can a slip of a girl understand my situation?' was another.

When it was pointed out that not all nurses were 21 but that more than a few of us are quite a bit older, the reaction was different.

'Yes, it would be good to have someone to talk to.'

One person with experience of nurses in the community said, 'Some are very good and do seem to be interested in patients as "whole" people; however, they are in the minority. Of nurses, 75% seem to be only interested in the presenting problem and how to alleviate that.'

Another person said, 'I think that it would be extremely kind of them to take an interest, it would certainly be helpful if it was provided.' Yet another said, 'Yes, but just giving advice is not enough – support is also important, yet that is often not forthcoming. They often tell you to lose weight, for example, but then don't provide the means to help you to do so.'

After explaining about the activities of living, the activity of sexuality was turned to and they were asked how they would feel about being assessed on that and, indeed, if they were aware of ever having been assessed on it.

All said that they had never been assessed on the activity of sexuality, never been asked questions about it, nor given advice.

One person said that when she attended the outpatients clinic after the birth of one of her children, the doctor asked her what contraceptive she used. She felt this to be none of the doctor's business and experienced it as an invasion of her privacy. 'Surely it is my business', she said. 'If I want information on contraception, I'll ask for it.'

Another woman said that following the removal of a breast lump it would have been very helpful if a nurse had discussed breast examination with her. Although she did examine her breasts regularly, the appearance of the lump had made her anxious and she wondered if it could have been detected sooner. 'I would probably be very embarrassed and I certainly would not start the conversation', she said, 'but nevertheless I think it would be a good thing.'

One woman related how she would very much have welcomed a nurse broaching the subject when she went into hospital for a laporoscopy. She was extremely anxious as there was a possibility of a malignancy, yet nobody talked to her about anything. Not only would she have welcomed nurses showing an interest in her as a person, she would also have welcomed more information on the actual procedure and the possible repercussions on her life if the result had been bad.

'That is all very well,' another woman said, 'but surely sexuality is not always relevant. If you go in for a varicose veins operation, for example, it is neither here nor there is it?'

'Actually it is,' said one. 'If it had been explained to me exactly what the effect on my appearance would be, I would not have agreed to that particular operation. Nobody told me that I would have all these scars on my legs. I definitely feel much less attractive sexually because of it.'

After that a discussion ensued on how sexuality is more than just sexual intercourse and how it is actually affected by quite a few physical as well as psychological problems.

'I suppose nurses can use their general observational skills and pick out quite a lot,' said one woman.

'Yes, that may well be, but what can they do about it?' said another. 'If I have a sexual problem, what can a nurse do?'

Activity 7

Read again the above conversation and pick out the relevant points. Do you feel people want nurses to care for them holistically? What is it patients would like nurses to do with respect to the activity of sexuality? Do you have any suggestions about how we could provide the care that people want?

Discussion

One of the points that is clear from the above conversation is that, sadly, qualified nurses do not necessarily spend a great deal of time with patients, leaving the bulk of the work to others. However, where qualified nurses do spend time with patients, they have the potential to be very helpful. Particular areas where nurses were seen to have a role was in information-giving and explanation. The idea of holistic care was welcomed, although none of the women thought they had actually experienced it. General support was another issue they had not experienced but would very much have welcomed.

With regard to sexuality, it appears that this is an issue which needs to be very sensitively handled as its relevance to nursing care is not always immediately obvious. Also, in this age of HIV and AIDS, some people may be suspicious and worry (as one woman said) that nurses are trying to ascertain their sexual preference in order to find out if they might be HIV-positive. It is clear, therefore, that sexuality is an area where skills such as observation, listening and communication are extremely important. Nurses need to be generally sensitive to patients' needs, worries and anxieties in order to give them the help that they need. Chapter 6, on counselling, will look into those skills in more detail.

There is a vast body of knowledge about how illness affects all aspects of sexuality. Whatever the nature of the illness, it is likely that some part of people's sexuality is affected – often in ways that they do not expect. Also, people are often unsure as to what is and is not advisable regarding sexuality.

Krueger *et al.* (1979) asked 108 women undergoing a hysterectomy whether they would like nurses to discuss aspects of sexuality with them. Half of the patients indicated that they would welcome such a discussion, as they were often unsure about how the operation would affect them. However, only 11% of the women reported that nurses had actually done this. It is not clear whether the other half of the women were unwilling to discuss the topic with nurses or whether their needs had already been met in another way.

It is possible that the women who did not state that they would like nurses to discuss the topic with them did not see it as part of the nurse's role, as nurses are sometimes seen as being concerned mainly with physical tasks.

Wilson-Barnett and Batehup (1988) in a discussion of physical handicap and sexuality state: 'Obviously, the message for nurses is clear. Many patients seek to engage in sex, wish to talk about their problems and need encouragement and positive attitudes from professionals' (page 96). According to Wilson-Barnett and Batehup, many people would appreciate advice on when to resume sexual relations after surgery or a serious illness. They make the point that, as many patients may feel unsure about whether or not to mention it, nurses should take the initiative and provide information, advice and support as part of their normal care as 'the research evidence is clear that patients have this need' (page 97).

WHAT ARE THE IMPLICATIONS?

Now that the topic of sexuality has been looked at from the nurse's as well as the patient's point of view, let us look back at the two and see what the implications are for clinical practice.

Activity 8

What do you think? What are the implications of the discussion so far?

Discussion

If you now feel that the whole field is rather daunting, you are in good company. It is precisely because the topic of sexuality is often not addressed sufficiently in nurse education and practice that the need for this book arose. However, we now know that illness in general, and some conditions in particular, affect sexuality. If we accept that nurses' remit involves care of the 'whole' person, then clearly we have a duty to address the issue.

You may have included in your list of implications that nurses need to have adequate and appropriate education and preparation. This preparation, you may feel, should be theoretical as well as practical. In order to include sexuality in our overall holistic care, we do need to see it practised – in other words we need role models. Supervised practice and mentorship schemes can be extremely valuable in helping nurses to acquire the essential skills required in observation, listening and other aspects of communication.

Another important implication you may have pointed out is that if nurses are to assess and help people with the activity of sexuality, they need to come to terms with their own sexuality first. Self-development and self-awareness should be a continuous process throughout nurses' education and should very much include an emphasis on awareness of their own sexuality.

Also, nurses should be aware of their limitations and know the extent and limits of their own personal capabilities, which are likely to develop over time and with experience. Constraints of service, regarding time, organization and staffing levels may, however, dictate that only a 'diagnosing' role can be played, referring more nitty-gritty problems (of whatever nature) over to specialists. Therefore we must ensure that those back-up services exist, that we know about them and that we have an established referral system. Some nurses may welcome a more specialized role. Indeed, there is much to be said for clinical specialists in every area who have undergone training in counselling as part of their general preparation.

REFERENCES

Krueger, J.C., Hassell, J., Coggins, D.B. *et al.* (1970) Relationship between nurse counselling and sexual adjustment after hysterectomy. *Nursing Research*, **28**(3), 145.

Roper, N., Logan, W. and Tierney, A. (1980) *The Elements of Nursing*, Churchill Livingstone, Edinburgh.

Seedhouse, D. (1988) *Ethics. The Heart of Heatlh Care*, John Wiley, Chichester, Sussex.

Wilson-Barnett, J. and Batehup, L. (1988) *Patient Problems. A research base for nursing care*, Scutari Press, London.

FURTHER READING

Johnstone, M.J. (1989) *Bio Ethics. A Nursing Perspective*, W.B. Saunders/Baillière Tindall, Eastbourne.

Mackie, J.L. (1977) *Ethics. Inventing Right and Wrong*, Penguin Books, Harmondsworth.

Rowson, R.H. (1990) *An Introduction to Ethics for Nurses*, Scutari Press, London.

Singer, P. (1979) *Practical Ethics*, Cambridge University Press.

Thompson, I.E., Melia, K.M. *et al* (1988) *Nursing Ethics*, Churchill Livingstone, Edinburgh.

Tschudin, V. (1986) *Ethics in Nursing. The Caring Relationship.* Heinemann Nursing, London.

CHAPTER 4

How women see the world

LEARNING OBJECTIVES

By the end of this chapter you should be able to discuss:

1. some views on how women experience the world;
2. the importance of relationships to women;
3. the role of sexuality in women's lives;
4. issues of dependency and illness.

> *'Because woman's work is never done and is underpaid or boring or repetitive and we're the first to get the sack and what we look like is more important than what we do and if we get raped it's our fault and if we get bashed we must have provoked it and if we raise our voices we're nagging bitches and if we enjoy sex we're nymphos and if we don't we're fridged (sic) and if we love women it's because we can't get a "real" man and if we ask our doctor too many questions we're neurotic and/or pushy and if we expect community care for children we're selfish and if we stand up for our rights we're aggressive and "unfeminine" and if we don't we're typical weak females and if we want to get married we're out to trap a man and if we don't we're unnatural and because we still can't get an adequate safe contraceptive but man can walk on the moon and if we can't cope or don't want a pregnancy we're made to feel guilty about abortion and . . . for lots of other reasons we are part of the women's liberation movement' (taken from a public toilet wall). ('Fridged' is the original spelling; we have not corrected it as it actually seems rather apt, and may have been intentional.)*

SOME VIEWS ON HOW WOMEN EXPERIENCE THE WORLD

A first impression is that this is an incredibly broad title. How could anyone say anything sensible about how women see the world? There are likely to be as many viewpoints as there are women. Yet people do make generalizations; we believe that certain views, ideas and characteristics apply more to women than they do to men.

Activity 1

Discuss the following question with a few people from various backgrounds and ages:

What are some commonly held generalizations about women's views of the world?

Discussion

The following views were collated.

Women want to have a man around, they like to be taken care of, they are passive and dependent, they are not really interested in the important issues in the world, preferring to occupy themselves with the minutiae of everyday life. Women are catty, they talk too much. Women are also warm, loving and like looking after children, men and anyone who needs it. Taking care of others is very much part of a woman's nature. Women do no longer want to be restricted to the home, they like to go out to work, have a career, earn a decent wage and be independent. Women like to enjoy themselves without necessarily being restricted by others.

Activity 2

There are a number of contrasting views in the above discussion. If you are a woman, how true do you feel some of these generalizations to be of you? Do they concur with your reality? Do you like them, are you indifferent to them, or do you find them offensive? If you are a man, how do these generalizations strike you? Which ones do you agree with?

Discussion

Whatever your reaction, there will be someone who disagrees with you. Women are many and views are many. However, generalizations do not appear simply in a vacuum, they are based on something. In other words, there must be a reason for these, rather than a completely different set of generalizations.

In fact, there are a number of commonly held stereotypes about women in society. They include the following seven examples; see if you recognize any of them.

The old maid

The old maid is easily recognized as she usually wears twinsets and pearls, or tailored suits. She tends to walk a great deal so wears no-nonsense, sensible shoes. Her skirt lengths are probably still just above the knee, having missed the various fashions for longer as well as shorter skirts. Fashion is not so much something she is uninterested in, it simply is something that has no relevance to her life.

She does, however, like to have her hair styled once a week by the same hairdresser her mother uses; she has been going there as long as she can remember, and these days has a blue rinse. She goes to church twice on Sundays, is a supporter of the Mothers' Union and other church-related organizations. In fact, she is a pillar of the local community and frequently writes to the local paper on many issues such as traffic noise, bad street lighting and the disgraceful state of the pavements with dogs fouling everywhere. She still lives with her elderly parents who are dependent upon her.

The feminist

The feminist is a woman who does not really care too much about her appearance and certainly does not dress up in feminine, frilly or sexy things as that would be pandering to men. She does not want to be judged on what she looks like but on who she is. She therefore tends to wear boilersuits, or men's jeans, with a shirt and waistcoat. She does not wear make-up and has short, cropped hair with long, dangling earrings.

She tends to be very serious, has no sense of humour whatsoever and has a short fuse on anything that appears to be a woman's issue. She is not interested in men, has no children and is probably a lesbian.

The housewife

The housewife is mostly found standing by the sink, with children, cats and dogs at her feet and budgies and a goldfish also somewhere around. If she is not in the kitchen she can be seen traipsing round the market loaded with shopping. She gets her husband's meal on the table as soon as he gets in from work or the pub and asks him about his day.

She has no outside interests as her life revolves around her home and children. She leaves all the big decisions and the financial affairs to her husband who is 'much better at that sort of thing'.

Business/career woman

The business or career woman is always very smartly dressed in expensive, well-styled suits with large shoulder pads, giving her a formidable appearance. She is perfectly groomed and never has a hair out of place. She is very confident, knows how to speak men's language and how to handle herself in a man's world. She is not married and owns a nice house or flat in the city, which is tastefully furnished and has all kinds of gadgets and labour-saving devices. Naturally, she never does any domestic work, employing a lady who 'does for her' three times a week. When she entertains she generally employs the services of a catering company. She does quite like men but will not allow them to rule her life, so she does have a boyfriend but tends to see him when it suits her.

The barmaid

The barmaid is found behind the bar in the local pub. She is voluptuous, and has lots and lots of dyed blonde hair which she back combs and wears in an elaborate style. She wears a great deal of make-up and favours tight sweaters which accentuate her ample bosom.

The barmaid is full of malapropisms such as 'the world is your lobster' or 'I'm absolutely ravishing' (instead of ravenous). She is extremely good hearted and although not one of the brightest, men tend to cry on her shoulder, particularly after a pint or ten. She does not really do much about this apart from say, 'There, there, have another drink, Charley.'

Good-time girl

The good-time girl is good looking and knows how to make the best of the features she has. She has glossy, long, blonde hair which she has cut every six weeks and long, perfectly formed, painted nails. She frequently visits her beautician, occasionally goes to a health farm and keeps herself in shape by aerobics, for which she has a variety of sexy outfits.

She enjoys life to the full, is always going out and has lots of casual male friends. She is well known at the local pub where she drinks five times a week, often before going off to a nightclub or disco. The good-time girl is in her 20s, and although marriage may be on the cards in the dim and distant future, she does not want to settle down yet for a long time to come. She likes to tease, and if she occasionally fails to come up with the goods she is called a prick- or cock-tease. Some men, usually ex-boyfriends, call her a ballbreaker. She may be a model or have a little job in advertising. She likes to take her holidays with the girls, when she generally enjoys herself and causes havoc. Last of all, she can look after herself.

Earth mother

The earth mother likes to wear a kaftan or long, floating Laura Ashley dresses. She burns joss sticks and bakes her own wholemeal bread every other day. She is vegetarian and one of her specialities is nut loaf. She and her husband have a small-holding and manage to live off the land.

She gave birth to her five children naturally and breast fed them all for at least a year. There is lots of wood and earthenware in the home as well as patchwork, which is one of her hobbies. Her kitchen is pine and has chunky cutlery and crockery from Habitat. She reads *The Guardian*, and relaxes over coffee in the morning doing the crossword. She supports Amnesty International, Greenpeace and Friends of the Earth, and has a job in the social sector or works part-time as a supply teacher, social worker or counsellor. She studies part-time with the Open University and shares much of the housework and childcare with her husband, who is of course a 'new man'.

There are, of course, more commonly held generalizations of women than are portrayed here. It may be useful to reflect for a moment and see what images come to mind.

Activity 3

Stereotypes aside, there are similarities between women's lives, particularly if they are wives and mothers. However, there are also many differences. What factors do you think might influence how an individual woman would see her life?

Discussion

We are all social beings. As soon as we are born, we are taken into a particular family, culture and nationality, and the socialization process begins. Social class, education, values, expectations, role models, financial status, age, appearance, nationality and culture, as well as a woman's physical state of health, all play a part.

As is implicit in Chapter 1 on the history of sexuality, women's and men's lives have undergone many changes over the centuries. In some parts of the world change is slower than others. The lives of peasant women in South America or India, for example, have probably changed very little. Most of their time is spent having babies and looking after their children as well as other members of the family. In addition, such a woman probably pulls her weight working on the land or taking part in some other activity by which the family earns its subsistence.

In Great Britain and other Western countries, however, women's lives have changed considerably in the last 100 years or so. The reasons for this are many. There have been and continue to be many social, economic, political and ideological changes which affect everybody's lives, women included.

As far as women are concerned, their lives have been influenced considerably by the various feminist movements, which started with the liberals in the nineteenth century and were followed by the suffragettes and the feminists of our own time.

Activity 4

It is sometimes said that we now live in a post-feminist age and that women are totally equal. To what extent do you think this is so?

Discussion

Friedan, a liberal feminist, wrote in 1963 that women's inequality was due to a 'feminine mystique' which was not based on reality and the purpose of which was to keep women at home (Friedan, 1982). In order to achieve full equality, according to Friedan, it was not sufficient to have equal educational, economic or civil rights, as women were often not in a position to benefit from these rights. In order to rectify the inequality balance, further reproductive rights were necessary, such as abortion, maternity leave and nurseries, which would enable women to work outside the home. Friedan's 'feminine mystique' was very much based on the white, middle-class housewife whose life, having achieved material satisfaction, nevertheless was devoid of meaningful goals.

Friedan's solution to women's lack of meaning, work outside the home, has not, however, resulted in equality for women. In many ways women's lives have become harder than before, because of the 'superwoman syndrome'. Although they had taken on board the solution to their sense of meaninglessness, women as well as men still clung to the feminine ideal of home and family, resulting in many women working a double-shift.

In the 1980s Friedan realized that the liberal solution of equal rights had considered only one half of the population and had left out men. In *The Second Stage* (Friedan, 1981), she argues that the 'superwoman syndrome' is counterproductive and symptomatic of the 'feminist mystique' which failed to value female 'fulfilment through love, nurture, home' (Friedan, 1981), but regarded efficiency as the ultimate goal. The solution, according to Friedan, is for men and women to participate equally in the home and to share everything equally, both possibly working part-time. An obvious criticism of this rather idealist solution is that it is feasible only for those earning good salaries; at the lower end of the social scale, both men and women work full-time out of necessity, not out of choice.

This later work by Friedan is an example of a new conciliatory rather than separatist feminist approach, which seeks to understand men and work with them. Tannen (1992), for example, in an effort to improve communication between the sexes, has written about the very different way in which men and women use language, which can lead to a great deal of misunderstanding. Jeffers (1989) uses a cognitive psychological approach and urges women to be less negative towards men and realize that their lives are not necessarily problem-free either. She points out that 'equality is more than anything state of mind' (p. 243) and 'does not come without responsibility' (p. 225).

As Nowinski (1989) points out, equality is a very important aspect of people's relationships and affects their sexual experience a great deal.

WOMEN AND RELATIONSHIPS

Activity 5

For this activity get together with some friends and discuss the following:

- What do men talk about with their friends?
- What do women talk about with their friends?

Is there a difference? If so, why is this, and what reasons could there be?

Discussion

It appears that when women get together they do talk about different things than men. Men tend to talk about sport and politics, whereas women like to discuss the things that go on in their lives. According to the linguist Tannen (1989) the reasons why men do not usually talk about personal issues is not because they are not interested in each other. It is because men's relationships are structured basically in terms of hierarchy and dominance. Women, on the other hand, are not usually concerned with dominance but with connection. Tannen gives many examples of how this is equally true for little three-year-old girls as it is for adult women.

Although some feminists would have us think otherwise, men and women **are** different. They are different physically, physiologically, emotionally and sexually. It is not clear to what extent these differences are inherent or acquired, the nature–nurture debate has gone on for a long time, and depending where one stands on the scale, different emphasis is placed on genes or socialization. However, it is true to say that whatever inherent differences do exist, they are enhanced greatly by the different ways in which men and women are socialized. People behave very differently to a little girl than they do to a boy. Girls are told they are pretty, must not get dirty or be rough and must be 'good little girls'. However, boys are encouraged to engage in rough and tumble, and if a boy shows interest in things normally associated with girls, such as dolls or prams, the chances are that he will be ridiculed. Although girls are not discouraged to the same extent to refrain from playing with toys normally associated with boys, such as cars or guns, they are not normally encouraged to do so.

Once children go to school peer group pressure further develops the socialization process. Although many teachers are not aware of it and sometimes resent the idea, it has been suggested that they behave rather differently towards the boys than to the girls in their classes.

Given the different ways in which boys and girls are brought up and the different expectations that people have of them, it is surprising that men and women still do manage to get on and understand each other. However, there is also a great deal of misunderstanding; women are often at a loss to understand why men behave the way they do and *vice versa*.

Why are men and women socialized differently?

Why is it that men and women are socialized so differently? We know that it happens, but why is it, what is the cause? According to Eisler (1988) things have not always been this way. She says that in the faraway past there was a period when men and women were truly equal. In her book, *The Chalice and the Blade*, she argues that whereas our society lives by aggression and dominance ('the blade'), this early society's symbol was 'the chalice'. This was a goddess-oriented culture which revered the qualities of love, nurturance and compassion for men as well as women. The creation and nurturing of life was seen as of prime importance, and consequently women were recognized as having an important role, and both men and women were encouraged to feel and express love and sexuality. This peace-loving civilization was, however, captured and eventually replaced by warlike tribes, the Kurgans, who lived by war, and for whom aggression and violence were a way of life. The earlier equality and mutual respect between men and women disappeared, with men of necessity developing their aggressive traits at the expense of their softer side of feelings and emotions. As men were much occupied with war and associated activities, women became responsible primarily for the rearing of the children and for the general nurturance of those members of society who needed it. Thus society was transformed dramatically and whereas men and women had initially been very close, now an ever-widening gulf was created between them.

As men and women's roles were so different now, they had to be socialized differently in order to function in their respective roles of warrior and carer. In today's society most men do not necessarily have to be involved with the army or fight in a war, although sadly there has been much increase in wars and particularly civil wars in the last few years. However, our society is structured to a great extent by what Eisler calls 'the blade'. The qualities that are valued in a man are independence, assertiveness, aggression, self-assurance and capability. It is not the done thing for men to show their feelings, rather they are expected to be in control of them and appear strong and unemotional.

Psychoanalytic theories

Of course, this is not to say that men do not have feelings, but that they are expected to keep them covered up. According to psychoanalytic theories, such as Eichenbaum and Orbach (1983), boys suffer a significant loss early in childhood when they realize they are not like their mother but quite different. Somehow they realize that they are to become like their father, who is, however, often much less in evidence. Consequently, many young boys are hurt and bewildered and learn to overcome this early trauma by burying their hurt. Whether or not one accepts the psychoanalytical view, it is true that many men are divorced from their feelings. Not only do they not express them because this would be frowned upon, but often they are genuinely not in touch with the feelings they do have. The only emotions that men are allowed, indeed encouraged, to express are anger and aggression, hence the sometimes (to women) incomprehensible scenes at sporting events.

Women sense the woundedness of men, sense their loss and often are attracted by the idea that they are the one to heal this particular man, and get through to him by the sheer power of their love. Examples in literature of this strong, silent but wounded man are Heathcliff in *Wuthering Heights*, and Mr Rochester in *Jane Eyre*. However, often the very things that attract women are also the cause of the eventual break-up of the relationship. If women are unable to somehow get through to the man and get him to express his emotions, at least on a regular basis, they get frustrated, hurt and angry and think the man does not love them and does not care. This is not necessarily the case; it is just that such a man does not know how to express his love.

Because men are not encouraged to be concerned with feelings, they tend to talk about things and events outside themselves – sport, politics, world events and so on. As Kramer and Dunaway (1991) put it, they are 'masters of the outer world'. Women, on the other hand, have never had to suppress their feelings because they do not suffer the early hurt caused by separation from the mother that boys have. On the contrary, according to Eichenbaum and Orbach (1983), they realize from an early age that they are like their mother and retain a close emotional tie with her.

As women are socialized to be nurturing and take care of people, they are in touch with the 'inner world' (Kramer and Dunaway, 1991). In terms of biology and history, this makes sense. With men engaged in hunting for food or defending the tribe against attack, women had to take care of their offspring, as well as the men, if the tribe was to survive. Caring for their chilren left women vulnerable, and therefore their survival was dependent on being protected by a man. Being able to attract a man was therefore of vital importance, especially as men's primary criterion for choosing a woman is often said to be her physical attractiveness (Kramer and Dunaway, 1991). Seen in this light it makes sense to socialize girls into the importance of being good little girls who look pretty; it is all a matter of survival. However, having attracted a man, it became equally important to be able to keep that man. In order to survive, women therefore developed nurturing and relationship skills.

Material vs emotional aspects

Ironically, the man best able to protect an individual woman would be the one who had most successfully been socialized into his role.

In other words the stronger and more aggressive a man was, the more likely he would be to be able to protect his family, therefore the more likely a woman would be to choose him. So it made sense in terms of survival for women to become attracted to men who were masculine and strong. In our society this means that many women tend to be attracted to powerful and successful men. Ironically, the more successfully a man has assimilated these aspects of his role, the less likely he is to be in touch with his softer side and the less likely a woman is to get emotional satisfaction from her relationship with such a man. Thus such a man is well able to provide for his wife and family materially, but the relationship is oten lacking emotionally. The more successful, dominant and aggressive the man, the more likely he is to be divorced from his feelings and the less likely he is able to understand what women want emotionally. In other words, the more his success in the outer world, the less success there is in his personal life.

So women have been programmed out of necessity to be attracted to macho men who are good providers, but who do not have much to give them in terms of closeness and intimacy. This being the case, women have come to rely very much on each other for emotional support. Most women have a network of close friends with whom they discuss what goes on in each other's lives, in other words, they discuss the 'inner world'. Men, too, rely on women for emotional support as they are not socialized to give it to each other. Indeed, to admit to each other that they have such needs would be a declaration of failure as a man. As is discussed in Chapter 5, on 'how men see the world', male relationships are very much structured in terms of dominance and hierarchy. Any sign of weakness, and emotions and feelings are seen as weaknesses, would therefore place them low down in the hierarchy.

As women are not concerned with hierarchy and dominance but with connection, men are safe to talk to women about personal issues without losing face. Traditionally, women have provided an oasis for a man where he can rest from the struggle in the outer world. Men's socialization does not let them get too involved, though; they both fear and desire a close relationship with a woman, creating a 'push me–pull you' dynamic. As soon as he feels he is getting in too deep, a man will pull back a little, until he feels too far away, or until he has a particular problem or emotional need, when he will again seek closer contact. As close emotional involvement is not a problem for most women, they do not understand this 'push me–pull you' dynamic and often get very hurt and bewildered by it. 'Does he love me or is he just using me for sex and comfort?' many women ask themselves. In fact, the issue of love versus sex lies at the heart of many relationship problems, as will be seen later.

It is not entirely true that women have not had to suppress any emotions; there is one they are not encouraged to express – anger. Anger, of course, is the one emotion which it is all right for men to have.

ANGER

Scenario

Chris went to a counsellor because she was confused by the fact that whereas she had always been a calm and easy-going person, just recently she had started to have bursts of quite unreasonable anger. After the latest episode she decided that she needed help as she was confused as to what was happening and was afraid she might do something she would regret.

The event that brought her to Jenny, the counsellor, happened one Friday evening. She had arranged to meet Frank, her boyfriend, in the pub after which they would go to the theatre, for which she had the tickets. When she got to the pub at the arranged time, Frank was not there, which was unusual, as he was normally very punctual. Some of Frank's friends were there and they said, 'What are you doing here, Chris? Frank has gone away for the weekend to that football match with a few of the others.' 'No, he has not,' Chris said. 'He has arranged to meet me here; we are going to the theatre.' 'Yes, I know that,' said Bob, 'He was here earlier and told us. It was all rather a spur-of-the-moment decision and he asked me to pass the message on to you. He said he'll ring you when he gets back.'

Chris did not believe it at first, but time went on, and half an hour later Frank still had not turned up. 'Honestly,' Bob said, 'I am not having you on, it is true, he has gone, ask the others.' Chris did and, yes, everybody agreed, Frank had gone away for the weekend with a few mates to see their team play an important match. Chris was now getting rather upset, and although she tried not to show it, apparently her face said enough. 'I'll just wait another ten minutes,' she thought to herself, 'and if he does not show up, I suppose it must be true.' Chris felt very upset, they had just gone through a rocky patch in their relationship, but were beginning to work things out. Now, she felt, all was finished and she had no other option than to break it off once and for all.

Suddenly, just as she was thinking of leaving, Frank walked in, full of apologies. He had had a particularly busy day at work and had simply fallen asleep. While she was relieved and very happy to see him she felt extremely angry with his friends. She was so angry that it made her afraid and she took care not to show it. Over the next few days the episode played on her mind, she just could not get rid of her anger. Chris realized that her reaction had to do with other factors; she thought she had finally found a good relationship after a very unhappy marriage and various short relationships which usually ended by the men letting her down in one way or another, or so she felt. Chris went to see Jenny as she just could not get the pub episode out of her mind, and it was beginning to drive a wedge between Frank and herself. She felt hurt by his failure to sympathize with her and side with his friends instead. 'It's only a wind-up', he said. 'What's happened to your sense of humour?'

Chris told Jenny that she was consumed by anger. 'I wanted to smash their faces in, I wanted to really hurt them.' She felt very frightened by these emotions as she realized they were way out of proportion to the incident. Also, she was not normally an angry person. With Jenny's help Chris came to understand that the pub joke was only one incident and just happened to trigger the anger which had been building up throughout her life. Very early on she had felt betrayed by her mother, who was rather inadequate and more interested in herself than her children and ultimately left the family to live with another man. Chris met James at the age of 22 and at first she thought she was happy. James was good looking, strong and told her that he loved her and how he only wanted what was best for her and would always go along with whatever she wanted. However, James changed almost as soon as they were married, informing her that as his wife he expected her to dress and behave in a certain dignified way. On the third day of their honeymoon, as she told Jenny, she dressed for dinner in an outfit specially bought for the occasion. It had been quite expensive and she knew she looked good. James took one look at her and said, 'You are not wearing that, other men will think ''She's a bit of all right'', and as my wife that is not on.' Chris changed her dress, feeling very confused and hurt. After all, she had dressed up to be desirable to James, not other men. But she clutched her hurt to herself. It was the first of many occasions and set the pattern of their marriage: James laying down the law, and Chris, in her eagerness to make a success of her marriage and not to follow her mother's example, swallowing her hurt and strenuously trying to fit James's idea of the perfect wife.

However, the harder she tried, the more demanding James became, until she could stand it no longer and filed for divorce. Jenny helped Chris to get in touch with her anger towards her mother as well as James and made her feel it was justified. She helped her vent her anger in a safe and controlled way, so that it no longer soured her relationship with Frank. After a while she felt ready to confront his friends and told them calmly, but clearly, that winding people up in order to have a laugh might seem funny at the time, but is actually very cruel, and can only have negative consequences. Although they apologis-ed, Chris was not sure to what extent her words were taken on board, but she felt much happier with herself. In a way, rather than letting other people control her emotions, she had regained her power and was able to use it. In fact, they all had a good laugh about it as Chris was now able to see the funny side of it too.

Chris's story is an example of what happens to many women. As men are out of touch with many of their feelings, so women are often out of touch with their anger. Anger is such an unacceptable emotion for many women that not only can they not express and show it to others, they hide it even from themselves, allowing it to grow and grow. This is what happened to Chris. From early childhood onwards, the anger had been building up in her, and suppressing it uncon-sciously had the effect of a pressure cooker. At some point something had to go, the anger could not be held in any longer.

Activity 6

Why should it not be acceptable for women to express anger? What could the possible reasons be?

First think about this yourself and then discuss it with a number of men as well as women.

Discussion

In saying that women are not encouraged to express anger it is not implied that they do not possess this emotion. It is just that they often have to suppress it, either consciously or subconsciously. This is because, in historical terms, anger was not likely to foster the har-monious and nurturing relationship a woman was trying to create with her mate. For a woman to express her anger with her mate would be a dangerous thing to do as her very survival depended on him. Also, as the man had all the power, there was actually very little to be achieved by it. Consequently, even today, women have very little experience with the expression of anger. Yet in terms of their every-day lives, many women are very angry, and men sense it and are bewildered by it. Women's anger probably plays a large role in the current high divorce rate; the majority of petitions are brought by women against men.

Although men and women's experience and expression of emotion supplement each other, because they are so different it is often the cause of much frustration and misunderstanding. Men often accuse women of being over-sensitive or over-emotional, with women accusing men of being cold and insensitive. Because women have little experience of anger they are often afraid of it and try to avoid causing their partner to be angry with them. When things go wrong women often look to themselves first, wondering if they are to blame. Because of this readiness to take blame, men may take out their problems, which initially had nothing to do with their wives, on them and, in a way, make them the scape-goats.

The different ways in which men and women handle emotion is evident from the following two scenarios.

Scenario

Bruce was always telling Rita 'not to raise her voice' and 'not to become emotional'. Showing signs of anger as well as upset were both frowned upon by him. Rita never did understand why the same rule did not apply to Bruce. When angry he would raise his voice and make his feelings known in no uncertain terms. When Rita pointed out that he was being emotional, Bruce denied this vigorously and said that he was merely bringing home a point.

Activity 7

Which dynamics are at play here? What is going on? Why do Bruce and Rita behave the way they do?

Discussion

Anger is often the only emotion men are encouraged to express. However, in Bruce's case he did not recognize it as an emotion. As far as he was concerned he was merely making a point. He had to make the point forcibly in order to get through to Rita, but he was sure that that was all he was doing.

Bruce was brought up in a male-dominated household. Apart from a baby sister who arrived when he was a teenager, Bruce had four brothers. Like many men, Bruce had been discouraged from boyhood onwards from showing emotion. Whenever Rita did become excited or upset he thought this rather unseemly and saw it as a sign of weakness, which, coming from a largely male household, he regarded as very embarrassing.

At the same time, although it is much more acceptable for women to express how they feel, the one emotion they are discouraged from expressing is anger. Consequently women often suppress their anger until they can do so no longer and it literally explodes, which is what happened with Rita.

Scenario

Jim is a marketing manager for a large international firm. His is a very busy job and he often works until eight or nine o'clock at night. At home he does not talk much to his wife Cindy; he comes home to relax and to unwind. Talking about work to Cindy would be like taking his work home, he says, and this he does not want to do. Generally, he is too tired to talk about much else and is quite content to leave the organization of the house and children to Cindy. Cindy, for her part, after having been at home with her two young children, looks forward to Jim coming home. However, she is becoming increasingly frustrated by the lack of communication between them and, as far as she is concerned, Jim does not seem to be very interested in either her or the children. She is very hurt and angry about this and lately has started to go to a number of evening classes. Consequently, she is often not there when Jim comes home, which is beginning to cause problems between them. Lately, Cindy has also lost interest in sex as she feels that is all Jim really wants her for. One evening, after a particularly bad row, they decide to seek outside help in an attempt to save their marriage.

Discussion

Jim and Cindy's story is very common and due to a large extent to the different ways in which men and women communicate. Men regard being committed to a woman and spending time with her as evidence that he cares about her. A woman, however, does not always realize that and wants a much closer relationship. Just being together is not enough, it is the quality of the time together that is important for women.

Unfortunately, men are often very uncomfortable by such close intimacy and see it as a sign that a woman wants to control, engulf or dominate them. This is understandable, as men's relationships are very much structured in terms of hierarchy and domination (see Chapter 5). All the woman wants to do, however, is connect; certainly in Cindy's case, domination was the last thing on her mind.

It was stated earlier that women do not express their anger, or that they have little experience in doing do. This is not entirely true. It is just that women express their anger in different ways than men. They do it less directly. Instead of confronting the issue and stating clearly how they feel, women may instead withdraw from the relationship, become less available, do less for the man, be less supportive and so on. Often, when a woman is angry about something, she will assume that the man will realize she is angry because she is not behaving in her usual way. However, men who are not used to this expression of anger, do not understand and may think she is just in 'bad humour' or a 'bad mood'. Often men see such a bad mood as evidence that women are over-emotional creatures, who are not always to be taken totally seriously, and they assume that the mood will blow over of its own accord. In other words, they do not necessarily think there is a reason for the bad mood, it is just something that women are prone to.

For her part, the woman gets even more frustrated and angry because her partner fails to pick up her anger signals. As far as she is concerned, it is perfectly clear what the matter is, and the man's failure to understand is seen as a sign that he is uninterested in her as a person and does not love her. And so the vicious circle of hurt and misunderstanding starts.

Expecting the impossible

Things are often made worse because so much is invested these days in man–woman relationships. With the demise of the extended family, couples are very much thrown upon each other. They are often unable to discuss things with other members of the family, and other family members are not around to pick up danger signals, give advice or smooth things over. Also, the high divorce rate notwithstanding, popular culture leads people to expect almost the impossible from relationships. Often couples look to each other for the satisfaction of their every need, physical, social, emotional, intellectual, financial, spiritual and sexual. Clearly, this is a very high burden to place on any relationship. Just imagine going for a job interview and being told you have to be all this for one person, would you take the job? However, because that is the expectation, that is what people think they should have. Women in particular, with the importance they place on relationships and connectedness, are often bitterly disappointed when their relationship does not give them the closeness, intimacy and togetherness they desire.

In fact, currently men as well as women are very confused and disappointed. We all have high expectations, but know at the same time that our relationships have a very high chance of failure. Also, because there have been so many changes in society recently we do not really know what is happening and what we should expect anymore. We are, as it were, in a state of transition, moving from one type of society and one type of relationshp to another. Because we are no longer in one situation and have not yet arrived at the other, we feel caught between the wall and the ship, trying to grasp at things which do not always prove fruitful.

In a way the women's movement has raised women's expectations, or rather it has shown them a way of life outside home and family. As girls now have the opportunity to be educated to the same level as boys, it no longer makes sense to expect them not to use that education, but to fit straight into the traditional role of nurturing wife and mother. Also, because our society has opened up a great deal through transport and mass media, women as well as men are much more aware of what goes on in the world outside their own environment, enlarging their world view and expectations. Women now are educated to have a job, which in many cases is more than just a little job to fill in time, or to earn a bit of extra money. For many women it provides independence and is often their only source of income. Married couples, too, often rely on their dual income in order to make ends meet.

So these days women very much pull their weight and are an established part of the labour force. Of course, there are still some occupations which are predominantly female, such as nursing, or male, such as engineering. However, inroads are made all the time and, in theory at any rate, a girl should be able to make her choice from any occupation at all.

Problems at home

So, having achieved to a large extent equality in the workplace, things often fall down in the home. Although there are exceptions, women are often expected to do the bulk of the housework, cooking and childcare, with the man very much taking a back seat. Why should this be so? Looking at the way in which relationships between men and women developed, it is not surprising. For thousands of years men have been the main providers, with women taking the responsibility of nurturing and childcare. To a large extent this traditional state of affairs still feels natural to many men, and also to some women. Indeed, even the women who resent having to do a double-shift, at work and at home, still comply with the traditional view – or they would not do it. Many women, no matter how well educated, or in how important a job, feel guilty. They feel guilty because they are not full-time mothers and housekeepers, but at the same time resent the fact that they do feel guilty. Women who choose to stay at home with their children, on the other hand, often also feel guilty as they are not doing what many other women do – combining two jobs, work and family. It is almost as if women are in a double-bind situation, damned if they do and damned if they do not. No wonder many women are confused and unclear as to exactly what they should be doing. All they know is that they try their very best but are exhausted all the time. At the same time there is this man, who thinks this is all a normal state of affairs, who goes to work and then comes home expecting to be looked after by her.

Men, for their part, are also often quite bewildered and think women do not really know what they want. They were brought up to believe that women are there to look after men, as they saw their mothers look after their fathers. Being looked after by a woman is for many men very much a right once they get married. Many, even well-educated, men see the role of the husband as that of the bread-winner and main provider, with the work of the wife very much taking second place. That this is so is demonstrated by the fact that if a man's job necessitates him moving town, it is expected as a matter of course that his wife will follow him. The other way round, a husband follow-ing his wife, is a much rarer event. Thus the job of the man still takes priority over that of the woman. Despite equal opportunities, it is often the case that men earn more than women, so it makes economic sense to regard men's jobs as being more important. When the wife earns an equal amount or even more than her husband, this can often give rise to problems in their relationship as the man feels undermined in his role as provider which, to him, is still his main function.

A certain unfairness?

So, given that the man still sees his primary role as provider for the family, it follows that when he comes home after a day's work he regards his day as finished, he had done his bit. The fact that his wife is still cooking and doing things in the home is only natural, that is part of her role. Some men realize that there is a certain unfairness in this and 'help out'. They may do the washing up or put the children in the bath. However, couples (as in the earth mother – new man stereotype) who share everything totally equally, without the wife asking the man to do specific things, are still very rare.

In a way, women are lucky. As there is not the same societal embargo on the expression of feelings, they are able to ask and receive help when they need it. Women like to discuss the smaller as well as larger frustrations and upsets as well as the joys of everyday life. As their men often appear uninterested or incapable of listening, women turn to their women friends for solace, comfort and sympathy. However, whereas this does help them, women are also disappointed that their men are unavailable to them emotionally. What they really want is to be close to the person with whom they live and have a relationship. In a way they often wonder – turning around the famous phrase from *My Fair Lady* – why can't a man be more like a woman? As a result women are, on the whole, healthier and live on average longer than men.

WOMEN AND SEXUALITY

Activity 8

Before going any further, please answer the following questions:

- What did your mother/father tell you about sex?
- Who told you about sex?
- What did they tell you?
- With whom do you talk about sex?
- What do you talk about?
- What for you is included in the term sexuality?

Discussion

These same questions were asked of 45 women, aged between 20 and 40, with mean age of 29. The following is a discussion of the questions asked.

What did your mother/father tell you about sex?

Thirty-eight of the 45 women said their parents told them nothing or very little. Only one person said her mother was very open about sex and that she felt happy to discuss whatever she wanted to know.

Seven people discussed menstruation, two having a baby, two contraception, one the male erection, and two were given a book to read.

Who told you about sex?

Quite a few people learned about sex from several sources. The vast majority learned about sex from school friends (40), closely followed by sex education at school (17). Three learned from their mother, two from an aunt and five from an older brother or sister, with four people being enlightened by television programmes. One person mentioned that she worked it out for herself by watching the animals on the farm where she live, and two were helped by boyfriends.

What did they tell you?

Answers to this question were varied: menstruation (7); reproduction (11); contraception (6); intercourse (18); everything (3); own experiences (4); reproductive systems (3); sexually transmitted diseases (1); what they had read (1); terms used (proper and slang) (1); lots of 'facts' that were not true (2); jokes (1).

Two answers were anecdotal: 'beware of boy scouts', and 'men jump from wardrobes onto women with spread legs'. (One woman scrawled all over her questionnaire ' ----- off and mind your own business'!)

The remaining questions were concerned with people's current experience.

With whom do you talk about sex?

The majority of women discussed sex with their husband, partner or boyfriend (35), and 31 also discussed sex with their friends. In addition, discussions about sex took place with: colleagues (10); children (9); sisters (1); brother (1); parents (4); patients (3); general practitioner (1).

What do you talk about?

Answers to this question come under four categories: factual, quality, general and funny. Five people said they would discuss absolutely anything, no holds barred.

(a) Factual

This included issues of pregnancy, family planning, contraception (20 people), menstruation (5), AIDs, safe sex and homosexuality (13).

(b) Quality

This included discussions on likes, dislikes and needs (11 people), and practices, experimentation, positions, deviance, expectations and enjoyment (26).

(c) General

Two people said they talked about values and mores, with three people discussing personal relationships, love or infidelity, and one person talked about fantasies.

(d) Jokes
Six people said they told jokes or talked about funny situations.

From the results it is clear that the majority talked about the actual nitty-gritty of their sexual experience. In other words, many women felt able to discuss fairly intimate details of their lives – usually with their friends. The factual discussions usually referred to discussions with children.

Finally, 39 women also answered the question 'What for you is included in the term "sexuality"?'

What for you is included in the term 'sexuality'?

Appearance (dress, make-up, looking good) (21); gender (5); feeling attractive to opposite sex (6); love-making, sex (4); relationships, love, caring (6); the way my partner makes me feel (loved, cared for, attractive, wanted) (1); morals, values (1); courtesy (1); being me as a woman (1); humour (1).

Out of the 39 women, only four actually mentioned sexual activity, the majority being concerned with appearance or feeling attractive. Only six of the answers related to relationships *per se*, without necessarily placing the emphasis on sex.

A woman's appearance

Although this was a very small group of women, it does emphasize how important a woman's appearance is thought to be. In terms of the above discussion, with men being attracted primarily by what a woman looks like, this is not surprising. Women know that they are very much judged by the way they look, hence the fortunes made by the fashion and make-up industry. Whereas it is not true that women dress and look in a certain way with the particular purpose of being attractive to men, looking and feeling attractive is very much a part of being a woman. It is bound up with how a woman feels about herself and how she feels herself perceived by others, women as well as men.

Men sometimes scoff at women's preoccupation with their appearance, and see it as an indication of not having to take them seriously as they are not really interested in the important things in life. However, this is somewhat disingenuous, as men like to be seen with an attractive woman. The more attractive the woman they are with, the more their own status among other men is enhanced. Women instinctively know this and therefore try to fulfil their part of the bargain. Of course, most of these dynamics are below a level of conscious awareness. Another dynamic which happens is that people tend to feel attracted by people they perceive to be of a similar level of attractiveness. Although it is true to say that women are not attracted primarily by a man's appearance, it is not correct to say that the way the man looks is not important to her. In terms of survival, as was seen earlier, a woman looks for a man who is strong, can protect her physically and is likely to be a good provider. Thus, clearly, a man with a good physique or a man who somehow exudes masculinity may be attractive to her as he is likely to be strong. However, with the demise of the hunter–gatherer societies, being able to provide these days is also associated with material wealth or intellectual prowess. Thus some women are attracted by the outward trappings of material wealth – good clothes, flashy cars or a string of professional qualifications. Hence the not uncommon sight of a very wealthy, but not particularly attractive, man with a very beautiful, perhaps much younger, woman on his arm.

Love and sex

So men and women place different values and priorities on what attracts them to each other. The message that our culture often gives through television soap operas, romantic novels and popular songs is that men have a high sex drive, which they cannot always control. Whereas women are now seen as interested in sex too, they are primarily interested in love. Sex without love is not usually desired on a long-term basis for most women.

What is the source of these views? Is it true that men and women view love and sex differently, or do they ultimately want the same thing? According to Jeffers (1989) many women as well as men are unhappy with the way things are at present. Many men are confused and do not understand what women want. Women, too, are often not happy, and feel very alone. When women get together, they tend to talk about personal issues, which often involve men. Because women are often frustrated in their relationships with men, they use the opportunity to complain. Statements such as 'Do you know what Jim did yesterday?' or, 'You wouldn't believe what Gary said ... ' all sound only too familiar. Putting men down is a favourite pastime for many women. 'Just like a man', 'Don't ever rely on a man/ask a man to do something', 'All men are the same', 'Men are useless', are all typical examples.

In a way, women use each other to relieve their frustrations about the way things are. It is not necessarily that they dislike men so much, it is just that they are hurt and disappointed because men often seem selfish and uninterested in them as people. The way in which our society has developed is partly to blame for this; we now put a tremendous burden on our relationships. As stated earlier, with the demise of the extended family, couples are thrown together and look to each other for fulfilment of their every need, physical, financial, emotional and sexual. Having the responsibility for someone else's happiness and the satisfaction of all their wants, needs and desires is frightening, and also doomed to failure. At no time in the past did people expect that much of each other in their relationships, as the extended family ensured that there were always plenty of other people around.

Due to the way in which we are socialized, women are often better off than men. Right from the word go it is all right for women to express their feelings, to cry if they are upset or to express doubt or fear if they are feeling insecure or afraid. On the other hand, men are given the message from a very early age that they must be strong and not show their emotions. 'Big boys don't cry', 'Don't be a cry-baby' and 'Don't behave like a girl', are the things boys have said to them if they show signs of being upset.

Scenario

Liz and Andy had been seeing each other for nine months. It had been a case of instant sexual attraction and they saw each other constantly. Liz was 35, Andy 29, so both had had previous relationships. In fact, Liz had been married for four years to a man who turned out to be very domineering and mentally unstable.

Right from the beginning Liz was unhappy in the marriage, and ultimately it ended in divorce. She was now rather cagey about relationships, but deep down wanted one that was going to last. She also worried that time was beginning to run out for her to have a family. Liz had enough experience to realize that mutual sexual attraction can feel very much like love, and she resisted for a long time the idea that it might be anything else.

Andy, too, had been married, and his relationship had also ended in divorce, but he had two young children whom he saw a few times a week. Andy freely admitted that he was 'a bit of a lad' and found it difficult to stick to one woman at a time. He did not really see anything wrong with casual affairs as long as the main lady in his life did not find out. However, his marriage breakdown was not due to other women, but to incompatibility. They had been very young, 19, when they married and simply grew apart. Andy was very fond of Liz and hoped the relationship would continue. He was not, however, looking to settle down or start a family. In fact, as far as he was concerned, the relationship was mainly based on sexual attraction and, as he says, he was quite happy to settle for lust.

Liz, although initially in agreement with this, knew that her feelings had changed from sexual attraction to love. Although the sexual part of the relationship was very important to her, ultimately it would not last if there was no love.

Liz and Andy are a typical example of the way in which men and women tend to see relationships and sexuality. Whereas both men and women look for love as well as sex, for women the emphasis is on love, for men on sex. In other words, casual relationships apart, women need to love and feel loved in order to function sexually, whereas for men this is not necessarily the case.

In order to have a lasting, happy relationship, however, mutual love and a good sex life are important. Many relationships run into problems because of the different way in which men and women view love and sex.

The 'double standard'

There is also the issue of the 'double standard' or 'double morality'. Notwithstanding the changes that have taken place recently in our society regarding sexual mores, it is still the case that it is more acceptable for a man to have many sexual partners than for a woman. A woman who is very active sexually and has many different partners is called a 'nymphomaniac'; the very word suggests that there is something wrong with her. It is definitely a term of disapproval. The male equivalent of nymphomania is officially 'satyriasis'; however, this term is not in common usage and most people have never heard of it. A very sexually active man is called 'a bit of a lad', or 'a right ram', which are not terms of disapproval. Rather, they express a certain grudging admiration and approval. For those with an academic bent, it is interesting to note that the word 'satyriasis' is based on 'satyr', a creature from Greek mythology, which was half-man and half-ram. Clearly, the expression 'a right ram' does ultimately have the same root as the word 'nymphomaniac', a nymph also being a creature from Greek mythology.

Traditionally, women were not supposed to be all that interested in sex, particularly not in the nineteenth century, hence the expression 'Lie back and think of England'. Since the advent of efficient methods of birth control such as the contraceptive pill, which took away the fear of pregnancy, the 'sexual revolution' has taken place. Women realized that they do enjoy sex much more than was traditionally supposed, it is just that in the past women often held back for fear of getting pregnant. Not only was it very much frowned upon to have a child out of wedlock, but married women, too, did not really want to have a child every year of their child-bearing years.

So, in theory at any rate, women are now free to have sex and enjoy it whenever they want to. The fear of HIV and AIDS has changed this somewhat, but this issue is the same for men and women. However,

the loosening of acceptable sexual behaviour for women has not come
without its problems.

Activity 9

Discuss the following issues with some people. How do men and
women relate to each other sexually at present? What codes of
behaviour do exist, and are there differences for men and women?
What, at present, are the problems related to sexual behaviour?

Despite the contraceptive pill, the illegitimacy rate has greatly
increased, although this is also due to the much-reduced stigma
attached to unmarried mothers. Some young girls in particular may
feel pressurized into having sex before they are ready. In the past they
could say no and use the fear of pregnancy as an excuse. Now,
however, that excuse has been removed, and a young woman may
be hard pressed to give a reason for not wanting to have sex. The
media also give the message that everybody is 'doing it' all the time,
sometimes on a very casual basis, which may lead young people to
think that this is the way it must be.

It is an interesting fact, however, that although women are matur-
ing physically earlier and earlier, and are therefore capable of having
sexual relations and becoming pregnant in their very early teens or
even earlier, sheer sexual enjoyment often comes much later for
women. Many women do not get into their peak sexually until well
into their 30s and 40s. There are various possible reasons for this. They
may have brought up their family and are therefore less worn out by
the strains of the 'double-shfit'; their marriage may have ended in
divorce, leading them to explore the excitement of new relationships;
their greater maturity may mean that they exercise greater choice, that
is, they have sex only with those men they really want to be with;
they are making up for lost time, not having had a chance in their
early years. There are probably as many reasons as there are women,
but it does indicate that women are capable of having and enjoying
sex far more than had been supposed in the last century.

Love and respect

However, despite the fact that older women are often able to enjoy
sex more for its own sake than their younger sisters, it is true to say

that eventually most women want a relationship that is not based just on sexual attraction. Even if the initial attraction between people is purely physical, in order to remain sexually responsive, a woman needs to feel that a man loves and respects her and is interested in her as an individual. In other words, she wants a close, intimate relationship, in which the partners talk to each other and share their feelings. Unfortunately, this is precisely what men are often not very good at.

Many men have problems expressing love and affection and are able to do so only through the medium of sex. Eventually this leads to the woman feeling used and unappreciated and causes her to stop enjoying sex with this particular man. It is an unfortunate fact that much of today's unhappiness between men and women is not necessarily due to people not loving each other enough, but to the basic differences between the way in which they express this love.

Men are often very hurt and surprised when their wives file for divorce. 'I had no idea that things were that bad,' said Bruce when Rita instigated divorce proceedings. 'We've had our ups and downs – doesn't everybody? – but we were OK in between.'

Bruce did not realise that Rita just hugged all hurt and disappointment to her until it had grown so large that it seemed pointless to carry on. As far as she was concerned nothing was ever resolved and nothing ever really changed. Whenever they did have a talk she felt that Bruce did not really mean it, but only went through the motions, and that they were just papering over the cracks. This is because Rita did not think that Bruce ever really said what he meant or how he felt.

All his problems at work were usually taken out on her, something he never admitted to because he did not realize he was doing it. Bruce thought that he had a genuine reason to complain when the house was not tidy or his meal was not ready on time. Because he was so divorced from his feelings, he did not realize that his failure to get promotion and his frustration at work were the real reasons for his discontentment.

His upbringing had also led him to expect perfection in the home, as his mother had waited on his father hand and foot. To him this was therefore a natural state of affairs. Rita, who had had a very different upbringing, resented this expectation and did not comply. She was an intelligent woman with many interests and saw this insistence of Bruce on an immaculate home and meals at certain times as ridiculous and an attempt by him to control her completely. Although initially she tried to comply for the sake of peace and because she loved him, Bruce always somehow found reason to complain, so she gave up. Both saw each other's behaviour as an indication that they were unloved, and things went from bad to worse until they were beyond repair.

Unfortunately, Bruce and Rita's story is only too typical. If they had gone for help in the early stages, they could have been helped to see that the differences in their upbringing and expectations caused the difficulties, not a lack of love, of which there was plenty in the beginning. However, by the time Rita filed for divorce she had stopped loving Bruce a long time ago, and they had not had sex for months. Although Bruce suggested belatedly that they should seek outside help, as far as Rita was concerned it was far too late and the marriage ended.

ISSUES OF DEPENDENCY AND ILLNESS

Many marriages and relationships run into problems because of a lack of intimacy. Often it is an accumulation of little things which, over time, grow into a wall of anger and resentment. Little disappointments are kept hidden and the hurt accumulates. The result is that there is a lack of openness and closeness, a lack of trust.

Sometimes couples go on like this for years. On the surface everything is fine. Sometimes they may not even realize themselves how shallow their relationship has become. Sooner or later, however, the gulf between them will become too wide to ignore any longer. One or both partners may lose interest in sex, or start an affair with someone else. The lack of closeness in a relationship is really shown up and problems are brought to the surface if one of the partners gets ill.

Illness may have a number of effects. It is possible that it will help couples to look at their relationship and decide that they do love and need each other, so illness can help to bring people closer together. It can also have the opposite effect. If the lack of trust and closeness has decreased to such an extent that it is practically non-existent, illness can be an intolerable strain.

How do women react to illness?

Activity 10

Find six of your colleagues and discuss the following situation.

The area where you work is very busy at the moment and is understaffed by three people, due to maternity leave, holidays and study leave, respectively. This morning you wake up feeling unwell with a sore throat and a headache. What do you do?

Discussion

The chances are that you decide to work anyway because to stay at home would make you feel guilty. Somehow it does not feel right to be ill, your function is to look after people, not to be ill yourself. This reaction by nurses, most of whom are women, is very much rooted in women's general experience and socialization. According to psychoanalytical theory, the behaviour of women in our society is regulated by repressed unconscious thought, which is itself based upon infantile sexuality (Kovel, 1981). Psychoanalytical theory, as developed by Freud, stated that girls become aware at the age of four that they are not boys as they do not have a penis. Both girls and boys regard the lack of a penis as a sign that girls are incomplete. Normally, girls' desire for a penis becomes transmuted to the desire for a baby. However, sometimes penis envy may develop, which manifests itself by women's jealousy; jealousy of men's higher status and wider opportunities. Thus, within Freudian terms, feminism is a consequence of pathological development.

Eichenbaum and Orbach (1983), however, dispute this view of women's sexuality and state that they have found no evidence that women regard themselves as incomplete or that they fantasise about a penis being transformed into a baby. According to Eichenbaum and Orbach (1983) it would be just as feasible (and incorrect) to say that boys suffer from breast envy as they will never be able to develop breasts or have a baby.

The last two decades have seen increasing criticism of psychoanalytical theory. It is now believed that several 'case histories' on which the theory is based were actually Freud's own dreams and fantasies while under the influence of cocaine. However, Freudian theory has been extremely influential to the extent of some of his concepts – such as the Oedipus complex, the castration complex or penis envy – having become part of normal everyday language.

Although Eichenbaum and Orbach (1983) reject Freud's view of women's psychological development as being linked firmly to early sexuality, they do agree that early experiences are important. Their theory is therefore essentially developmental. However, contrary to Freud, they see women's development occurring much earlier than the age of four or five, and state that as soon as a baby is born, there is a subtle difference in the way it is treated, depending on whether it is a boy or a girl. Overtly this difference is demonstrated by the traditional blue clothes for boys and pink for girls.

According to Eichenbaum and Orbach (1983) women's development is part of an ever-perpetuating cycle. As in patriarchal society, women are second-class citizens (Miller, 1976), they have to defer to men and always put their own needs second. Mothers, consciously or subconsciously, teach their daughters from an early age to look after others as part of the preparation to be a second-class citizen. The relationship between mothers and daughters is not straightforward but ambivalent and subject to 'push–pull' dynamics. As part of their development women learn to hide and repress their own needs or, as Eichenbaum and Orbach call it, their 'little girl selves'. However, when a woman has a daughter, the 'little girl' in her identifies with her daughter and projects her own needs onto her.

As the mother has learnt to hide her 'little girl self' she teaches her daughter to do the same by not meeting her needs (push dynamic). The daughter experiences this as rejection and attempts to become separate from the mother. This attempt at separation is felt by the mother as a 'loss', therefore she does not help her daughter to become separate, but instead sends out messages of need (pull dynamic). (Figure 4.1)

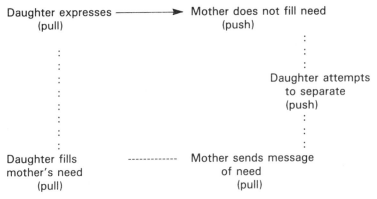

Figure 4.1 Push–pull dynamics.

As she had already taught her daughter to repress her own needs in favour of those of others, the daughter is compelled to meet her mother's needs. Thus the mother becomes the daughter's first child. The result of the confused and dual messages women receive throughout their childhood results in the lack of a strong separate sense of self. A consequence of the 'jagged attachment' with the mother is a lack of personal boundaries and a profound feeling of insecurity and low self-esteem. One way in which women's lack of personal boundaries may be demonstrated physically is by the fact that women (as well as men) approach women to a far closer distance than they do men (Weitz, 1979).

Our male-dominated, patriarchal society does have implications for men, too, as under the guise of masculinity they are often distanced from their own emotions (Tolson, 1982). According to Tolson, man's development is also characterized by conflicting dynamics in that, to a boy, masculinity is both attractive and threatening. This simultaneous distance and attraction results in a permanent emotional tension and uncertainty which leads to a compulsive need for recognition and reward. However, concealed within the 'rat race' of modern life is men's emotional insecurity and emptiness. Although men may not realize their own emotional needs, women do sense men's insecurity and attempt to meet their needs. Thus men continue to function because of the support of women; however, this support is largely unrecognized.

As women learn from an early age not to expect to have their needs met, but instead to look after others, their needs go underground and become repressed. Subconsciously many women have deep feelings of neediness, isolation, depression, anger, disappointment and rejection. They often lack self-esteem and have a fundamental feeling of insecurity. The failure to have their needs met causes women to fear their needs and feel ashamed of them. They feel that if their needs were to come out in the open, they would be insatiable, uncontrollable and ugly. Consequently, women actively, albeit subconsciously, suppress these needs as a defence mechanism in the same way that, as seen earlier, they suppress anger. This defence mechanism has a dual role and is felt to protect both the self and others.

By not exposing their needs, women protect themselves by avoiding hurt and humiliation. As women's needs and little girl selves are felt to be ugly, unlovable and unacceptable, their repression protects others from being confronted with them. However, although defence mechanisms may be a form of self-protection, they can also prevent care and help from coming in and thus be self-destructive. In developing defences to protect them from anticipated hurt, women also prevent themselves from being supported.

The nursing profession offers a good example of the development of these defence mechanisms. It has been argued that women often transform their needs (Miller, 1976) and that those who enter nursing may do so to fill a need within themselves to be nurtured. When we are faced with sick and dying patients we feel often woefully inadequate and unable to give the patient the support he or she needs. Being brought face to face with human suffering makes a new nurse feel vulnerable and aware of her own needs and shortcomings. In order to cope with the situation she may therefore develop a fairly sophisticated 'professional manner' of being busy and unavailable for support.

This 'professional distance' from patients protects nurses from the suffering around them. However, as nursing colleagues often have constructed similar defence mechanisms, they may receive no help when they themselves need it. There is fairly substantial body of evidence which shows that, despite their professional distance, nurses are affected by dying patients and bereaved relatives. However, nurses are not expected to express this hurt and are often supposed to cope without any help whatsoever. Thus, patients, relatives' and nurses' needs all continue to remain unmet.

Eichenbaum and Orbach's theory of women's psychological development explains why women feel so isolated, unworthy and empty (1983). E.M. Forster put women's experience very succinctly in his well-known phrase 'panic and emptiness' which seemed to engulf women at inopportune and unexpected moments (*Howards End*). A similar panic confronted the heroine in *Passage to India* also by E.M. Forster. Unfortunately, the film version a few years ago failed to understand this and changed the entire meaning of the book by assuming the heroine's panic was due to fear of her own sexuality. Forster's solution to the panic and emptiness was to 'only connect', as in connecting with others at a deeper level women can lose their isolation and become whole.

Although women look to husbands and children for fulfilment of their incomplete selves, they do not really believe that anyone will let them be close and separate simultaneously. Women are therefore afraid that they may lose themselves and become merged with their partner. Thus their already shaky sense of self-identity is threatened even further. This fear of loss of self is not without grounds as in this society women are defined in terms of their husbands and children, and with any married couple the man is seen as the head of the household, and women's social class and standing is defined in terms of her husband's occupation. 'What does your husband do?', or 'How many children do you have?' are often the only type of questions ever asked of married women when, for example, attending a party or meeting people for the first time.

In addition, women are expected to give up their surname (and in this country sometimes even their first name) and be referred to as Mrs Joe Bloggs. Although these examples may be regarded as conventions only, they do embody fundamental values of patriarchal society and thus become absorbed in women's and men's innermost psyche.

Women's collective experience is one of 'countless put-downs by men' while continuing to support men, thus allowing them to play their dominant role (Tolson, 1982).

In their relationships with men, women's repressed needs tend to show up in a covert form. To pretend to be physically weak, unable to replace an electric plug or to understand how to fill in a tax form can be seen as a conscious or unconscious attempt to be taken care of. If the covertly expressed need is below the consciousness level it is probably due to 'learned helplessness' (Seligman, 1974). It is, however, also possible that women use the pretence of helplessness quite consciously to pay men back for always having their needs met. Thus they get 'one over' on men and slightly despise the men when they 'fall for it'. Another method women use to manipulate men to get what they want is by subtly planting an idea in a man's mind and then praising him when he expresses it as his idea. An example of this is the 'doctor–nurse game' whereby a nurse gets a doctor to prescribe the treatment that she wants without appearing to express an opinion (Stein, 1978).

Eichenbaum and Orbach have come under attack from some feminists who see the theory as somehow blaming women for the position they are in. This is incorrect. Eichenbaum and Orbach do not blame, they merely point out a cycle which occurs as a consequence of women's position in a patriarchal society. As all men and women are influenced by the society in which they live, the concept of blame in this context is inappropriate. Eichenbaum and Orbach attempt to clarify the way things appear to be. It is essential to have a clear picture of a situation before attempting to help people who are hurt by it.

So what happens when a woman gets ill? Often she simply has no time to be ill and carries on regardless. If she has to be admitted to hospital she worries about her husband and children, she feels guilty and unentitled to be ill.

Activity 11

Think of some particular women patients. How did they react? What was their prevailing mood? What did they talk about?

Discussion

The atmosphere on a female ward is usually quite different from a male ward. Women tend to be worried, talk to each other about their problems and may try to help each other by talking and listening, while men often laugh and joke but often take care not to confront the main issues that bother them.

However, for men as well as women, their 'need' is very close below the surface. A mature experienced nurse, who is calm, exudes confidence and is able to pick up cues from the patients can help a great deal, simply by being there and really listening. It is by listening, using the active skills discussed Chapter 6 on counselling, that nurses are able to enter the patient's world, empathize and get a 'feel' for what they are going through.

True empathic understanding, without judging or labelling, will be of tremendous benefit to the patient, who will feel valued and cared for. Feeling that there are people who really want to understand, and who care enough to take the time to listen, is a very important part of getting on the road to recovery, or coming to terms with whatever is going on. Chapter 6 will discuss how a variety of physical problems may affect people, particularly with regard to sexuality and how nurses may be able to help

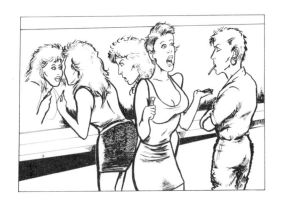

REFERENCES

Eichenbaum, L. and Orbach, S. (1983) *Understanding Women. An Expanded Version of Outside In–Inside Out*, Penguin, Harmondsworth.

Eisler, R. (1988) *The Chalice and the Blade. Our History, Our Future.* Harper & Row, San Francisco.

Friedan, B. (1981) *The Second Stage*, Summit Books, New York.

Friedan, B. (1982) (originally pub. 1963) *The Feminine Mystique*, Penguin, Harmondsworth.

Jeffers, S. (1989) *Opening Our Hearts to Men. Taking Charge of Our Lives and Creating a Love That Works*, Piatkus, London.

Kovel, J. (1981) *A Complete Guide to Therapy*, Pelican, Harmondsworth.

Kramer, J. and Dunaway, D. (1991) *Why Men Don't Get Enough Sex and Women Don't Get Enough Love*, Virgin, London.

Miller, J.H. (1976) *Towards A New Psychology of Women*, Penguin, Harmondsworth.

Nowinski, J.(1989) *A Lifelong Love Affair. Keeping Sexual Desire Alive in Your Relationship*, Thorsons, Wellingborough.

Seligman, M.E.P. (1974) Depression and learned helplessness, in *The Psychology of Depression: Contemporary Theory and Research* (eds H.J. Freeman and M. Katz), Winston–Wiley, Washington.

Stein, I. (1978) The doctor–nurse game, in *Readings in the Sociology of Nursing* (eds R. Dingwall and J. McIntosh), Churchill Livingstone, Edinburgh.

Tannen, D. (1992) *You Just Don't Understand. Women and Men in Conversation*, Virago Press, London.

Tolson, A. (1982) *The Limits of Masculinity*, Tavistock, London.
Weitz, S. (1979) *Nonverbal Communication*, Oxford University Press, New York.

FURTHER READING

Friday, N. (1991) *Women on Top. How Real Life Has Changed Women's Sexual Fantasies*, Hutchinson, London.
Henderson, J. (1987) *The Lover Within. Opening to Energy in Sexual Practice*, Station Hill Press, Barrytown, New York.
Litvinoff, S. (1991) *The Relate Guide to Better Relationships. Practical Ways to Make Your Love Last, From the Experts in Marriage Guidance*, Ebury Press, London.
Zweig, C. (1991) *To Be a Woman. The Birth of the Conscious Feminine*, Mandala, London.

How men see the world

LEARNING OBJECTIVES

After reading this chapter you should be able to:

1. discuss some views on how men experience the world;
2. discuss the importance of relationships to men;
3. identify the role of sexuality in men's lives;
4. discuss how men react to illness and dependency.

MEN – THE STEREOTYPES

Men like everything to go their way, and it's not their fault if it doesn't.
First-year nursing student

To do this chapter heading justice, a considerable number of men would need to be interviewed so that a collection of representative ideas could be presented. Such an idea is, of course, beyond the scope of this book. However, what is offered are some commonly occurring themes or stereotypes, for want of a better word. The stereotypes are presented as a common reference point from which discussions can, and should, take place. They are therefore not submitted as a definitive representation of men.

So, what type of men exist? What are the commonly occurring stereotypes in our society? The following are six possibilities.

The real man

A man who usually has a physical or active job, like a road worker or building worker. The type that shouts or whistles from the building scaffolding. He may also be found supporting the bar with his mates, giving every woman the once over, and making comments by cracking dirty jokes. It would appear that male bravado increases in direct proportion to alcohol. So the more alcohol he consumes, the more daring he becomes, egged on by his equally rowdy mates.

His personal hygiene and dress sense need attention, and he displays tattoos of varying size and description. He thinks women find him irresistible. Some attractive qualities would be his beer gut hanging over the front of his trousers while the cheeks of his bottom are glimpsed every time he bends down. In the back pocket of his trousers can usually be found a copy of *The Sun* newspaper, not for the news and views, but for the 'boobs'. To prove that he's 'one of the boys' he will get drunk and touch up women because he thinks they find him desirable, and they like it anyway. When they say 'no' they really mean 'yes'. He does not believe in equality among the sexes, and is of the opinion that a woman's place is in the home, looking after the children and doing the cooking. He has strong outside activities like football, and possibly belongs to a rugby or social club, where the beer is cheap. Surprisingly though, he always finds someone to marry him!

Mummy's boy

This man cannot, or does not, want to break free from home with his mum. He is about 30-plus years old, has never had a steady girlfriend, likes the quiet, peaceful life, home cooking and the routine, which has been his way of life since he can remember. A typical job would be a clerk for the local council. He can be found every Saturday doing the shopping with mum. This man has got a very strong hobby like stamp collecting or train spotting, from which he has a close and small circle of friends. He goes on holidays every year with his parents to Great Yarmouth or Anglesey. Any girlfriends would have to contend with, and come up to the same standard as, his mother. He will not spend his money frivolously and as a consequence will not be sporting the latest fashions. A plain, hand-knitted tank top, cords and a pair of sensible shoes will see constant wear.

The new man

Married, and happily so for the past 20 years. He has two children and a wife who is also his friend. They share responsibility for the running and upkeep of the home. It would not be out of character for this man to do the washing and ironing, and put the children to bed while his wife does pottery in night class. He would also encourage and support his wife in her career, seeing the relationship as an equal partnership. He would be sensitive to his wife's and children's feelings, and not too concerned about showing his caring and compassionate nature. His interests have political and ecological connotations – Greenpeace, anti-nuclear protests – and he is a subscriber to environmental friendly products. He is a keen gardener, and likes to keep fit with outdoor pursuits. The whole family goes swimming once a week. He believes in supporting his children's education, and will treat them as intelligent, free thinkers. He would not consider having an extra-marital affair, because the relationship with his wife provides all he needs. Besides, if he felt the need he would have probably discussed it with his wife.

The stud

This man is the lean, mean, bonking, dancing machine. He usually hangs out at discos, has blond hair, muscles and he knows/shows it. This man could also be known as a poser. He has good up-to-date fashion sense, and will spend as much time in the gents' toilet as the ladies do in theirs. He does not understand the meaning of a long, deep and meaningful relationship. If he does not get 'his' women into bed on the first date then he's off with somebody else who will come up with the goods. It is as if he has something to prove to his mates about how successful he is. He drives a flashy car, perhaps a Golf GTi. The car has such loud music pouring out of it that everybody looks as he drives past, fast. Young girls will swoon over him, while the older ones try to forget him. He may one day settle down and marry, but he will never be satisfied with one woman.

The gay man

Gay men can be divided into various stereotypes (Pickles, 1984).

- The closet queen. This person is gay but spends his whole life denying it. He may openly be disgusted at anything homosexual.
- The clone. Clones, as the word suggests, all look alike. They wear white T-shirts, lumberjack type shirts, jeans, boots and a thick moustache.
- The young gay man. He finds it difficult to fit into everyday life. He has his own circle of close friends and when he is with them he is completely different. He may have to live his life very carefully. Disclosing his true nature and feelings could be disastrous. His life at work or within the family is contradictory to how he feels.

It is becoming easier for gay men to 'come out' and not be ashamed about their sexuality. In the past few years there has been a number of role models for gay men to follow. Television has also played its part in desensitizing homosexual behaviour. Remember the first kiss between two men in prime time television – *Eastenders*? The gay man has a number of female friends who enjoy his friendship because they do not see him as a potential relationship or threat to their own sexuality. The lifestyle and generally sensitive nature of the gay man are also appealing to women. He has good dress sense, and tends to keep himself looking and smelling respectable. His relationships can be either tortuous or stable, the former being the most common. Some gay men can end up marrying, and do so to either escape their own sexuality or to fulfil the need to have a family.

The commonly held view of gay men is that they are effeminate and limp-wristed, spending all their time mincing around looking for men (Sanderson, 1989).

The married man

This man has been married for as many years as he has had affairs, although the unsuspecting woman who falls into his trap does not realize this until it is too late. He will have an outgoing personality and the gift of the gab, so that he can put you completely at ease. This man will initially treat women with great respect, and will wine and dine them until the romance starts to fail, and then small excuses start to occur. The woman will then start to suspect something is just not right, and will confront him. This leads to a nasty tearful scene, when he tells her that he did not want it to turn out this way, and he is sorry if he has hurt her. He will, of course, never leave his wife. This affair is short-lived until the next woman comes along, and the cycle is repeated. It is possibly the stability in this type of man that women find so attractive, plus the fact that he has had lots of practice.

These sterotypes are not true representations of the types of men in our society. There will, of course, be some men who from time to time fit into some or a number of categories. However, it is possible that after reading the above discussions, certain familiar images are recalled. If they are familiar to you, then this may add weight to the argument that stereotypes do serve a purpose. Or is it possible to generate more stereo-types of men? Before answering that question try the next activity.

Activity 1: Typical men

Make a list of about four men who you know. For example, husband, boyfriend, brother, uncle. For each of these write a list of words or statements that best describe their attitude to life. What characteristics do they show in relationships? How do they spend their time socially? Do they have firm views about par-ticular subjects or issues?

After making a list, can you identify any commonly occurring factors? Do any of them fit into the previously discussed stereotypes? Or can you make different headings to describe what you have found?

THE MAKING OF MEN

He's a big handsome boy, isn't he? My word, he looks like he's going to be a boxer or a footballer. Just like his dad, isn't he?
                                                              Visitor to a new baby

What happens to men to make them into the people they are? Are they born that way or does something happen while they're growing up? Certainly from the moment we are born we are socialized into the role society expects us to play for the gender we have been assigned. The opening quote is one of many commonly heard remarks that relate to the aspects of our gender. One of the first questions at birth is, 'Is it a boy or girl?' So from the moment we are born the gender role is, to a degree, set; we then have to learn how to behave according to our sex. Or do we learn? To what extent does genetic make-up make men the way they are? There are those that would argue that men behave the way they do out of biological necessity. They are driven by their genes. In order for their own genes to survive (which is of paramount importance), they must be passed on to the most appropriate female. Searching for the correct female is motivated by physical desire as well as biological mechanisms. The importance males attach to this could be related to their aggressive nature. To survive, and for the female to judge that the offspring will also survive, she needs to choose a male who is strong. Displaying this 'strongness' may mean being aggressive. Could this explain why some women feel attracted towards those men who lead a less than peaceful life. Whether this is true or not, it would be true to say that men are more aggressive. That is not to say that **all** men are aggressive, but when compared to women, more men than women are aggressive. This may be a consequence of the hunter–gatherer days in prehistoric times, where being tough meant survival (survival of the fittest).

If two newborn babies, one boy and one girl, were laid side by side there would be very obvious physical differences. Yet at that very early age there is no other obvious gender differences which identify one as a girl and the other as a boy. Babies are just babies – doing baby things. The movement from a baby to a boy and then a man (and similarly for girls) involves a process of learning, or social-ization. Early on in a baby's life they are described differently, even though such differences are not obvious nor the consequence of any behaviour. Boys tend to be described as tough, loud and big, while girls are described sweet, quiet and petite. Even if the true sex of the baby is not noticeable, people still behave in a way appropriate for the sex of the baby. In one experiment a number of mothers were observed interacting with a six-month-old baby called Beth. Their behaviour to this girl was typical: they smiled a lot, offered dolls for it to play with and thought the baby was 'sweet'. Similarly, another group of mothers were observed interacting with a six-month-old baby boy, Adam. Their responses to the boy were different from the girl. They thought the baby was strong and big, and offered a train as a toy for play. Yet Beth and Adam were actually the same baby, dressed differently for each occasion (Will *et al.*, 1976).

The degree to which or how a baby is socialized into its gender role will depend on a number of factors, such as class, culture, race, education and religion. Men growing up in a Jewish household will receive entirely different gender messages than a man growing up in a Indian home. Young Jewish men will go on to experience the world differently from young Indian men. Given this cultural and social disparity, it is easy to see how conflict may arise across cultures. Values, attitudes and behaviours will also be affected. To what degree depends on the extent of integration, and the naturaliza-tion of the family. These are important aspects to consider when dealing with patients from different ethnic backgrounds from the host country.

It becomes obvious that there are many ways in which a man may develop. Many influences could affect the final result. Yet in all this there appears to be some commonly occurring themes, especially within the Western culture. One would be the way in which men see women, while another is how men see their own sexuality.

MALE SEXUALITY

What are little girls made of? Sugar and spice and all things nice. What are little boys made of? Slugs and snails and puppy dogs tails.

It is worth mentioning at this point that the term 'sexuality' does not mean simply sex organs or the sexual act of intercourse. Sexuality has a wider remit than the purely physical. It is about how one sees and experiences the world, and how men fit into that world. Chapter 2 provides more discussion on this topic.

The first awareness of our own unique sexuality is the delight taken in exploring our physical being. Babies start to make sense of the world around them through the senses of taste, touch, hearing, sight and smell. Unfortunately, when these senses are turned onto the baby's own body, discouragement is all too common place. Young children are dissuaded from touching themselves. 'It's not nice to touch down there.' 'Leave it alone or it'll drop off if you keep touching it.' 'Don't do that, it's naughty.' These are a few of the common responses from most parents. Presumably parents react in this way because their own parents reacted in the same way. Or, as parents, they are not at ease in discussing sexual matters. So early attempts at understanding ourselves are met with obstruction. Learning that 'down there' is wrong, naughty and something to feel guilty about is taken on board very early on in life.

Correct and expected behaviour is another learned aspect of what being a male is about. Lessons that 'big boys don't cry' or 'Go on and stand up for yourself – be brave' are part of the process of becoming male. A consequence of such action is that very early on boys learn to suppress their natural sensitivity. Boys are taught to concentrate on getting results from action, with most of their play spent around activities – 'getting on with things', playing with cars, building things with blocks, discovering how things work. All these have an affect in directing the child's attention towards a more productive outlook on life. Girls, on the other hand, are allowed to express their sensitivity. Playing with dolls, making home, even enjoyment and delight are expressed. It is common and acceptable behaviour for girls to giggle, scream and be excitable. Next time you see children playing, take a moment to look at how they express themselves through play, and the toys they use. Of course it would be foolhardy to suggest that the gender learning discussed above is strictly adhered to. As our society changes, and our understanding about sexuality and gender develop, there will be a merging of ideas about what boys should do and what girls should do.

As children develop the factors influencing learning about gender roles increase. Children start going to school and therefore mix with other children. Television and books also affect how a growing child perceives his gender. Work which has examined children's books highlights clear differences in the gender roles they portray. Males tend to be depicted as adventurous, and involved in discovery and outdoor activities, which demand strength. Females are depicted as passive and confine themselves to domestic affairs (Weitzman *et al.* (1972), in Giddens (1989)).

Activity 2: Children's stories

Examine some of the commonly occurring children's books, fairytales and nursery rhymes. Take a moment to read through a number of the stories. Is it possible to identify different gender roles? What happens when you reverse the gender roles and the parts males and females play in the narrative?

Adults also play a part in enforcing the type of acceptable gender behaviour. Parents do this either through conscious effort and thought, or by unconscious role modelling. As the developing child grows and starts to make sense of the world, he/she is bombarded by messages from all directions; some are conscious, while others are subliminal.

By the time boys are in their early teens they have learnt a number of important issues. They start to move away from childish things, and how they play and what they play with changes. Their relationship with girls is also affected, and they start to prefer boys' company. It becomes increasingly important for them to be accepted by other boys of their age. It is during the early teens that boys start to move away from sensitive caring aspects, such as being kissed by auntie, crying after a fall and being frightened by spiders. Putting up a brave front on these matters is achieved with varying success; perhaps men are never really able to. What happens is that with varying degrees men tend to bury their sensitive nature. Some men will be able to suppress their feelings so deeply that they will not show. Others may experience real conflict between what they feel and desire inside and what is expected of them in terms of gender role. This potential conflict of feelings and resulting behaviour has implications when nursing men, and will be discussed later.

FROM A BOY TO A MAN

When and how this happens seems to be arbitrary. Adolescence is the term given to describe the transitional period from boy to man. Boys or young men move through stages in their development with varying speed and success. As a boy, you are under the control of an adult. As an adult, you have more freedom. So at its simplest, adolescence could be described as a shift in power. The movement from boyhood to manhood is not a clearly defined passage, unlike in other cultures where 'rites of passage' (as they are termed) make the distinction of when a boy becomes a man.

In Judaism the male has a barmitzvah at the age of 13 to mark the passage from boyhood to manhood. In mainstream Western culture, no rites of passage exist. Reaching and working through adolescence is therefore a trial and error procedure. Boys have to reject childish aspects of life and take up more masculine attributes. Achieving the status of adulthood can be traumatic. There will be times when boys feel vulnerable and confused about who and what they are becoming. To a large extent, boys have to work through this process alone; to ask for help and support would be a sign of weakness, unbecoming of a man. With varying success and absence of psychological trauma, the boy becomes a man.

BEING A MAN

Man's love is of man's life a thing apart
'Tis women's whole existence

Byron

Activity 3: It's a man's world

Try answering the following questions:

1. Is society geared or organized in such a way that it is better suited for men than for women?
2. Do men behave differently when with a group of other men compared to when they're on their own?
3. Is it easier for men to succeed in a career than women? If 'yes' why?
4. All men really want out of life is sex, whereas women want a loving lasting relationship.
5. Men don't really understand what it's like to be at home with the kids all day. They have it easy by going out to work.

Being a man is about being powerful; any model of masculinity has this as a component. This has problems because men do not always see themselves as powerful. The male adult world is made up of a hierarchy, which contains winners and losers. Men see the world more competitively than women, men being driven by some sort of innate desire to have power over others. These 'others' are usually women and children.

This rather dominant and perhaps ignorant view is not shared universally. There are signs that men are beginning to change in their outlook to life and to women, presenting society with a so-called 'new man' (see above). The 'new man' is not just an invention of the glossy magazine, but is the reclamation of what has always existed. Deep down men are sensitive, caring, nurturing people – it is just the effects of years of socialization that have made them into the people they are, or that society expects them to be. So the title 'new man' is a misnomer. Being and becoming a new man encompasses a number of principles.

1. Showing and talking about feelings are acceptable for a man.
2. Valuing and cultivating the relationship men have with women.
3. That the relationship men have with women is seen as equal.
4. That responsibilities are shared when caring for children.

Moving into a scenario where the above principles apply is threatening to men. It will take time and courage; but it should be remembered that the ideas are not about creating something new, rather they are about allowing aspects of man out (Harvey, 1991).

COMMUNICATION

Listen, Joan, this idea of you getting involved with Jackie, it involves money, and you're not experienced in handling money. Why don't you just concentrate on looking after the home, doing the housework, cooking and Tom, and that's your job done?

How often has the following expression been heard? 'He just doesn't understand what I mean.' It was George Eliot who said, 'We are all islands shouting lies to one another across seas of misunderstanding.' It would appear that on some occasions men and women experience tidal waves of mendacity. Tannen (1986, 1992) has devoted two books to the subject of misunderstandings of men and women in conversation. The book, *You Just Don't Understand. Women and Men in Conversation* (1992), details the essence of the problem – men and women experience different worlds, and describe that world with different words. Men tend to look at the world through the concepts of independence, aggressiveness, rationality and objectivity, while women look at the world through the concepts of intimacy, morality, passiveness and dependency. The concepts are poles apart; 'It is as if their life blood runs in different directions' (Tannen, 1992, p. 26).

Knowing this, is it any wonder that our communication styles are different? That we ever communicate anything would seem good luck rather than good judgement. When we apply these concepts to our health care system, a certain picture emerges. Doctors, the majority of whom are male, control the running of health care, while the majority of those delivering the health care are nurses, and are predominantly female. This means that female nurses have to overcome what is a male-dominated profession if they wish to become truly autonomous. Savage (1985) has discussed this aspect further.

Even everyday language has aspects of sexism in it. 'He's the best man for the job.' 'How many man-hours have we lost this week?' 'The average man in the street.' These three examples are by no means exhaustive, and it is not until one stops for a moment to consider it that one realizes how much of our language is male-orientated. The use of everyday language that has male connotations could be deemed similar to subliminal advertising, in which one acts in response to subconscious messages.

Activity 4: She says – he hears

This activity can be carried out as a group exercise or between two people, one male, one female. The males and females are separated by a short distance (so that each can be heard), each pair facing one another. The females then communicate the statements below to the male opposite. There is no need to say the statements in any particular way. In fact no inflections or stress on certain words should be made. The males are asked to make notes on **what the remark felt like to receive**. It is important not to write down what was actually said.

Females ...

1. Shall we go and see Jim and Carol tonight, I really miss their company?
2. How long will it take you to finish decorating the front room? I'd like to measure for curtains as soon as possible.
3. Would you like to call in at the next restaurant for a rest, after all, you've been driving a long time now?
4. You're not going out again, are you?
5. Are you having another drink?

After the females have finished, the males then take a turn and in the same manner as described above repeat the following statements:

Males ...

1. Oh, that's quite a nice dress.
2. Oh, you're wearing that dress, are you?
3. Do we have to go shopping now?
4. Why does it take you so long to get ready?
5. The lads are coming round tomorrow night; are you going out, or what?

As research for this chapter, the authors asked 48 nursing students (average age 22 years) to make a statement on the following question: 'How do men see the world?' On content analysis, the females (38) mentioned the following: dominance, authority, aggression, power, good job/career, money/rich, family, wife/girlfriends/partner, car, sex/lust, materialistic, and health. While the males (10) mentioned: love, to give love, protect/security, control/power, provide/breadwinner, career, money, good status/successful/fame, macho image, sex, marriage, home and flashy car. There is some common ground in respect of men being seen by both groups as having control or power. Good employment which gives security and promotion was another common denominator.

A CHANGING WORLD

In the last 20 years or so many changes have been seen to gender roles and their resulting effects on male sexuality: the growth of the feminist movement and the position women hold both in society and the workplace, for example. The assumption that men have power and control over women is fading fast. The changing economic climate together with widespread unemployment (three million at the time of writing) has lead to a decline in the traditional 'breadwinner' role. In some instances families have seen a role reversal, with the woman going out to work while the man stays at home with the children. The present society places great emphasis on materialism and ambition. The consequence of such a philosophy is the stress it causes when men do not achieve. Stress and related conditions can be compounded should the man be part of a peer group who share the same ideals.

Gay sexuality is being given a higher profile. More and more men are 'coming out' and talking about their true sexuality. This changes people's ideas about previously established models of male sexuality. Human immunodeficiency virus (HIV) and the resulting acquired immune deficiency syndrome (AIDS) have directly challenged men's sexual attitudes, values and behaviour. It is no longer considered a 'gay plague', and is growing faster in the heterosexual population than in the gay community. The disease is forcing men to reconsider their sometimes casual sexual behaviour of the past.

HOW DO MEN REACT TO ILLNESS?

One aspect of being a man is about being in control. It is about having power over oneself, and in varying degrees over other people. When men become ill they lose some of that power. The extent of power loss is relative to the illness or disease. In an effort to make this section meaningful, a number of scenarios are presented. They should highlight some of the problems and behaviours nurses may experience when men become ill. It should be noted there are no helping strategies offered to the problems, as these will be covered more fully in Chapters 6 and 7.

Scenario 1

Mr Beckett has been in hospital three days, after suffering a mild heart attack. He is a very busy man and works as a sales executive for a computer company. He is 45 years old and at the top of his profession. As for most heart problems, complete rest was indicated. Sally, an 18-year-old student nurse, was on her second ward, and had been allocated to care for Mr Beckett during her span of duty. It was during a bed bath that Mr Beckett took great umbrage at Sally's manner. He said she was too off-hand, giggly and unprofessional. Mr Beckett asked if somebody else could care for him.

Discussion

This scenario presents a number of reactions. First, Mr Beckett could be acting in this way because of a loss of control. It should be remembered that he is a sales executive and is used to making his own, and other people's decisions. Second, he may feel embarrassed about being bathed by such a young girl. He may identify Sally with someone within his own family, a daughter perhaps, and as such react to her in that way. Third, Sally may be acting that way because she is uneasy with the intimacy. She may also sense that Mr Beckett is embarrassed by the situation and tries to make light of her activities, but this is taken the wrong way.

Scenario 2

David has been on the medical ward for the last two months. He suffered a complex neurological problem which has caused loss of muscle control and therefore a degree of paralysis. He is now starting to recover slowly. He has a dutiful wife, Grace, and three children. During one of Grace's visits, David became very angry, raised his voice and swore at her. Grace left the ward in floods of tears. It transpired that David did not want his wife to visit so often, and he had lost his temper when she suggested bringing the children in to see him.

Discussion

David has had a long, protracted illness which has left him in a partially paralysed state. The extent and dependency of his illness will have affected his self-esteem. His role as a provider to his family will be affected. He may feel helpless in supporting his family, and sees his wife as taking over this role (role reversal). His role could also be affected in the future were the disease to return. The lengthy illness will have affected the relationship between David and his wife. It is important also to remember that the illness could be responsible for the outburst. David could also be concerned about how he looks to his children. He could be fearful that the children may be alarmed at the sight of his condition. His masculinity and role function have been compromised by the illness, an illness that has no physically apparent signs, like a broken leg or scars. This lack of observable disease does not allow for focusing. It is possibly more difficult to come to terms with an illness when there are no outward signs of its existence.

Scenario 3

Derek Jones is a 52-year-old bachelor, who has long standing diabetes. He is being cared for in the community. For the past six months Derek has had a leg ulcer which is not healing despite using various dressings. The dressings have to be changed every day, which means a district nurse calling. The district nurses find Derek very chatty, so much so that they find it difficult to get away. It was during a call that the district nurse noticed Derek irritating his wound by pushing a knitting needle down under the dressings. When the nurse questioned him he simply said that it was itching him. The wound was reassessed one month later and found not to be healing.

Discussion

It is not unusual for district nurses to see people in the community and know that part of their visit is for social reasons. Derek could be a person who looks forward to these visits. They may even be his only contact with a woman. The self-harm inflicted by pushing a knitting needle into his dressing could be a means of prolonging the visits. It is expected behaviour that all patients should want to get better; it is part of the sick role (Parsons, 1972). When a patient refuses to comply with treatment and has no desire to get well (particularly a man), it confuses the impetus of care.

Scenario 4

Ian is a 22-year-old suffering from cancer. For the past four months Ian has been visiting his local hospital for chemotherapy. The anti-cancer drugs have affected him in a number of ways: vomiting, nausea, listlessness and hair loss. It is this last aspect of the therapy that has caused Ian the most concern. Before his diagnosis Ian was very active; he would play football every weekend, and socialize most evenings. He has a longstanding girlfriend of three years. However, since his diagnosis Ian has basically become withdrawn and retreated into his 'shell'. He very rarely socializes, and the relationship with his girlfriend seems to be deteriorating.

Discussion

The subject of cancer and its nursing implications is huge. Whatever is written here will not do justice to the complexities of the disease. However, the reason for its inclusion in this section is to serve as a reminder that serious life-threatening illness can overshadow the patient's sexuality. Atwell (1984) suggests that there are three possible areas in which cancer may affect a person's sexuality.

1. Decline in sexual interest due to the psychological impact of cancer. This could be a factor with Ian's strained relationship with his girlfriend. He may fear that his abilities, be they physical or emotional, have been weakened by the disease.
2. Changes to body image due to treatment. Ian's hair loss has been the aspect of the treatment that has caused him most concern. Body image and appearance have become increasingly significant over the last 10 years. Vanity in men is as important as it is in women. Ian may feel that his appearance has been greatly affected.
3. Impotence due to treatment. This is an inability to attain and maintain penile erection. This could also be affecting Ian's sexual relationship with his girlfriend. There is a great deal of importance placed on the sexual act, particularly by young people. Ian was a very active social person, and has been exposed to peer pressure. Such peer pressure may have affected his perceptions of sexual role and performance.

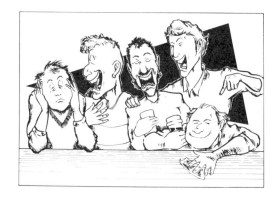

REFERENCES

Atwell, B.A. (1984) Sex and the cancer patient: an unspoken concern. *Patient Education and Counselling*, **5**, 3.

Harvey, I. (1991) Men's talk ... men's group. *Nursing Times*, **87** (26), 32–4.

Parsons, T. (1972) Definitions of health and illness in the light of American values and social structure, in *Patients, Physicians and Illness* (ed. J.E. Gartley), Free Press, London.

Pickles (1984) *Queens*, Quartet Books, London.

Sanderson, T. (1989) *How to be a Happy Homosexual. A Guide for Gay Men*, GMP, London.

Savage, J. (1985) *The Politics of Nursing*, William Heinemann Medical Books, London.

Tannen, D. (1986) *That's Not What I Meant! How Conversational Style Makes or Breaks Your Relations With Others*, Virago Press, London.

Tannen, D. (1992) *You Just Don't Understand. Women and Men in Conversation*, Virago Press, London.

Weitzman, L. *et al.* (1972) In Giddens, A. (1989) *Sociology*, Polity Press, London.

Will, J.P., Giddens, A. and Datan, N. (1976) Material behaviour and perceived sex of infant. *American Journal of Orthopsychiatry*, **46**, 162.

CHAPTER 6

Counselling skills

This chapter will explore what is involved in effective listening. The activities are designed to try out various forms of listening and to facilitate self-awareness on the part of the listener.

LEARNING OBJECTIVES

By the end of this chapter you should be able to:

1. explain what is meant by counselling;
2. identify factors which influence communication;
3. demonstrate effective listening skills;
4. recognize the need for further reading and practice;
5. recognize that self-awareness and personal development is a lifelong process.

HOW TO READ THIS CHAPTER

Listening is regarded as the most important of all communication skills. It seems easy but how many of us can honestly say that we are always really listening to what people try to tell us? The purpose of this chapter is therefore to explore exactly what is involved in 'listening'. Listening and counselling will be looked at from a general point of view. Chapter 7 will apply the skills discussed more specifically to the area of sexuality.

Like ethics, listening is very much an activity, and the best way to learn to listen effectively is by practising. This chapter is therefore structured around activities. They follow a logical sequence, so it is best to do the activity before carrying on reading.

It would not be a good idea to try to work through the whole chapter in one sitting, as the nature of the material necessitates a certain amount of reflection, consolidation and, in some cases, observation.

You may find it useful to come back to this chapter at a later date as the activities may be carried out at various levels. You may well find that you get something different out of an activity every time you carry it out. The way you use this chapter does not therefore have to be linear, you can back-track and go over what you have done before – albeit probably at a deeper level. You will probably be surprised at how much more you get out of an activity the second or third time; it will also help to consolidate what you have learned previously.

This is because of the 'microwave effect'. When a dish is taken out of the microwave, it must be left to stand for a while because the cooking process is continuing. In the same way you continue to process your experiences – either consciously or below the level of immediate awareness. That is why it sometimes helps to go and do something entirely different if you are trying to find the answer to a problem. The answer may then just 'pop up', seemingly out of the blue.

WHO CAN COUNSEL?

Practical counselling and helping skills are not the exclusive province of mastectomy counsellors or clinical psychologists. Whichever area of nursing you work in, it is likely that you already carry out a certain amount of counselling. You may find that you support people in your private life; your friend may look to you for help after a break-up with her boyfriend, for example, or your sister is distressed because of her child's illness.

There is nothing magic about counselling, it is something that we can all do – but there are ways that are more effective than others. This chapter is therefore a down-to-earth guide which may help you to further develop the skills you already have.

It is encouraging that more and more people in the caring professions now see the need for counselling training and are attending counselling courses, often in their own time. You may find that the skills you learn spill over into everyday life and make you generally more responsive and able to see someone else's point of view.

Most activities are to be done by at least two people. That is because if you want to practise listening, you have to have someone to listen to. So it would be good if two of you worked through this chapter together. If it is hard to find the time, you could make it a social occasion – have a bite to eat or a glass of wine, or both. There is no law that says you cannot. Go on, make learning fun!

WHAT IS COUNSELLING?

Activity 1

Pause for a minute and think about the following:

- What do you understand by the term counselling?
- What do you think your colleagues understand counselling to mean, or your boss, your teacher, doctors, the patients?

Jot down a few ideas and discuss them with a colleague.

Discussion

In 1978 the Royal College of Nursing set up a working party to look into counselling services. It was found that within nursing, counselling can mean anything from comforting, to giving information, to correcting and discipline. From the varying definitions and descriptions of the counselling process, the working party selected the following definition as the most helpful and relevant to nursing:

Counselling – a process through which one person helps another by purposeful conversation in an understanding atmosphere. It seeks to establish a helping relationship in which the one counselled can express his thoughts and feelings in such a way as to clarify his own situation, come to terms with some new experience, see his difficulty more objectively and so face his problem with less anxiety and tension. Its basic purpose is to assist the individual to make his own decision from among the choices available to him.

Royal College of Nursing (1978)

This rather lengthy definition may be shortened to: 'to enable the person to help himself' (Nurse, 1980).

It is this meaning which is implied from now on when the word counselling is mentioned.

WHAT IS INVOLVED IN COUNSELLING?

You may already have a good idea of some elements involved in counselling.

Activity 2

Spend a few minutes thinking about the things you feel play a part in counselling.

Jot down your thoughts. You could ask a partner to do the same and then compare your results.

Discussion

You probably surprised yourself with the variety of your answers. There are no good and bad answers, as there are a variety of approaches and ways of thinking about counselling.

You may have said that it involves a relationship, such as that between a nurse and a patient. Such a relationship may be characterized by genuineness, sensitivity to the patient's feelings, warmth and an absence of labelling or judging.

Alternatively, you may have concentrated on the skills involved; good communication skills, particularly non-verbal communication, such as eye contact, facial expression or body language are very important. Similarly, you may have pointed out the importance of being able to pick up a patient's non-verbal signals. Other skills include being able to ask open questions and really listen to what is being said.

Implicit in the definition of counselling given by the RCN (1978) is that, essentially, it involves self-help and personal responsibility. Linked to this is the idea of choice. We cannot tell someone else what to do; if we try, we may end up with egg on our face as invariably we choose what is right for us rather than what is right for the other person.

What we can do is help people to see the various options open to them and thus help them to perhaps become better choosers.

The approach we tend to use in nursing is based on humanistic psychology, which sees people as able to change themselves and change their lives, without having to continually carry the burden of the past or the conditioning of their environment (Burnard, 1987).

This is a marvellously liberating approach. It does not matter if you have made a mess of things, or, if it does matter, you do not have to go on suffering because of it. You are free to put it behind you – it is up to you. Helping people to see that is a very great gift to give them. But it may take time; it is not easy, and it requires a certain amount of courage. It may be easier to stick to our rigid ways of thinking, as to change may require us to take a good look at ourselves, and we may not always like what we see. We tend to judge each other, and our patients, all the time, but the person we judge the hardest is often ourself.

But we do not have to be so hard on ourselves. After all, we are all only human, none of us is superwoman or superman. Even the people who seem to stand out way above us have their weaknesses and are probably very uncertain inside. They just hide it better.

To be non-judgemental is therefore an important part of counselling. Who are we to judge anyway? It is extremely liberating to talk to someone and to know that you are accepted for what you are – good or bad – no-one is judging. Being accepted unconditionally by another person is a great help in becoming accepting of yourself. Too often we do our patients a disservice while thinking that we act in their best interests.

Activity 3

Mrs Evans, in hospital for the umpteenth time with exacerbation of her chronic bronchitis, but who still smokes 40 cigarettes a day, may get frequent tellings off. You may have come across similar situations where you thought you knew what was best for a patient. What did you do, and what happened?

Think about this for a few minutes. If you have time, it would be helpful to discuss your experiences with a colleague.

Discussion

Mrs Evans does not need to be told off. She probably feels bad enough about herself already. Rather, listen to Mrs Evans, find out how she sees the situation and what choices she feels are open to her. It never works trying to force people to do something anyway; the choice will have to be made by themselves.

ARE YOU LISTENING?

The ethos of holistic nursing, as seen in Chapter 3, requires that in addition to physical care, nurses also provide psychological and emotional support for patients. We are now much more aware of the close links between mental and physical well-being, and emotional support is therefore no longer considered a luxury.

Several studies have shown that patients who receive adequate emotional support actually recover more quickly (Bundy, 1989; Gruen, 1975; Mazzuca, 1982; Schlesinger, Mumford, Glass *et al.*, 1983). Therefore, within the current economic climate, it is actually becoming cost-effective to provide counselling training for nurses.

But how good are nurses at providing emotional support? Truax and Miller (1971) investigated scores of 13 occupational groups on empathy, warmth and genuineness – three qualities thought essential in the provision of support. They found that, along with manufacturing plant supervisors, registered nurses had the lowest scores.

Matthews (1962) asked 122 staff nurses in hospitals in California to respond to statements which they had to assume were put to them verbally by patients. Only eight nurses gave responses that would encourage the patients to enlarge on what they were experiencing. Matthews also found that nurses' ability to empathize with patients and see things from their point of view actually became less the longer they had been qualified.

Why should this be so? One reason may be that nurses are always so busy running around looking after people's physical needs and doing the one-hundred-and-one jobs that nurses do, that it is sometimes easier not to notice the patient's distress. The trouble is, after a while it becomes the norm and nurses no longer realize their shortcomings.

Activity 4

Think of times when you felt unable or inadequate to help a patient. What kind of problem was it? What made it difficult for you? It may be useful to discuss this with a colleague.

Discussion

Often it seems that nurses just do not know what to do, because they feel inadequately prepared for the things patients say to them. They simply do not know what kind of response would be helpful.

You may have thought of times when you did not know how to respond when a patient asked if she was dying. Perhaps you felt inadequate when Mrs Jones was in tears because her husband had just died. Or maybe you just didn't know how to respond to Mr Smith, who appeared so depressed since his stroke.

Activity 5

Can you think of occasions when you perhaps pretended not to hear a patient call or not to notice her distress?

- What made you pretend not to notice?
- What would have happened if you had noticed?
- Think about these questions for a few minutes.

Discussion

Because we do not know how to deal with patients' distress, we develop a shell and keep a 'professional' distance. This helps us to cope and keeps us going. But how much good is such 'professionalism' doing the patients?

The nursing process and approaches such as primary nursing necessitate us to become much more closely involved with patients than hitherto. Becoming more closely involved is likely to result in our becoming more aware of patients' emotional distress and worries.

Patients may look to us for support and it is therefore important that we feel confident in such a situation. However, providing emotional support is not easy and, until recently, has not really been taught in schools and colleges of nursing.

Some think that people who can provide emotional support are born that way, rather like good nurses. Most people, however, agree that there are certain skills involved, and, as with any skills, they can be learned.

Probably the most important skill of all is listening. 'Anyone can listen,' you may say. 'I do it all the time.' Yes, but do you? **How often do you really listen?**

Listening, in a counselling sense, is summed up by a lovely quote from the ancient Chinese philosopher Lao Tse:

It is as though he listened and such listening as his enfolds us in silence in which at last we begin to hear what we are meant to be.

The listening in this quote refers to a total awareness of everything that goes on when two people are together. If a nurse listens in this way, she can help patients to become listeners, too, and help them to listen to themselves, see themselves clearly and thus help themselves.

Helping patients to help themselves is what nursing is very much about these days. Gone are the days when the nurse did everything for a totally passive patient. Counselling also aims to help people to help themselves, so clearly nursing and counselling have much in common.

How can we learn the type of listening referred to by Lao Tse? Well, first of all, there is a simple exercise you can carry out, either by yourself or with others, wherever you are. Try it now.

Activity 6

Sit in a comfortable position with your back well supported. It is best to have both feet on the floor. Close your eyes. Become aware of your body, its weight on the chair, the feeling of your feet on the floor, and your clothes against your skin. Listen to your thoughts, feelings and emotions. Do not think about them or judge them; simply note them and let them go. After a minute or so, turn your attention outwards to any sounds that you can hear, both close by and far away.

Carry on this activity for approximately three or four minutes.

Discussion

How was that? What did you notice? What did you feel? What did you hear? Was it easy? Did you like the activity? If not, why not?

Sometimes we find it difficult to sit still. We are always so busy that it seems almost perverse to sit quietly for a few minutes. However, unless we learn to be quiet we cannot learn to really listen.

If you do this activity twice a day, you will find it easier and easier. You'll probably look forward to it as it is a marvellous way to unwind and recharge your batteries. After a few weeks you can do the activity with your eyes open, and 'listen' with your eyes, simply noting everything you see without passing judgement.

This listening activity is really an awareness exercise and should help to sharpen your powers of observation generally.

HOW TO LISTEN

Therapeutic listening really consists of three phases: (1) receiving and understanding; (2) communication of your understanding; and (3) an awareness in the other person that you have listened and understood. Clearly, used in this way, listening is rather wider than what we usually mean by the term.

To make things a little clearer it is necessary to discuss some theory; don't be put off by the jargon – nursing jargon is just as bad. Until this author became a nurse, he thought mobilizing had something to do with the army!

Barrett-Lennard (1981) calls listening 'facilitative relational empathy'. It sounds a mouthful, but what it means is that there is a relationship between two people, involving empathy on the part of the listener which facilitates the speaker to say more.

Using Barrett-Lennard's terminology (1981), the three phases of listening are:

- empathic listening;
- expressed empathy;
- received empathy.

Empathic listening is basically understanding what has been communicated, whereas expressed empathy is the communication of that understanding, which may be verbal as well as non-verbal. Received empathy is an awareness on the part of the other person (for example, the patient) of the expressed empathy. The whole process is really a continuous cycle, the 'empathy cycle' (Barrett-Lennard, 1981).

Listening involving empathic resonation includes seeing things from the other person's point of view, seeing the world from where he is standing, getting into his internal frame of reference.

To get into somebody's frame of reference, you need to listen to what they are saying just as much as to how they are saying it. You also need to be aware of any accompanying messages they are sending with their body.

Activity 7

Take the following phrase, for example: 'I don't really mind'. It can be said in a variety of ways. Try saying it in different ways with both your voice and your body. Then take turns with a partner at trying to say it in as many different ways as you can think of, altering your body language each time.

Can each of you pick up what the other is communicating? Can you get into her internal frame of reference?

Discussion

I can hear you think, 'If there is an internal frame of reference, there must also be an external frame of reference.' You are right, there is. If you stay in an external frame of reference you do not attempt to see things from the other person's point of view, but only from where you are standing. This is seen too often in nursing. Nurses do not see things in the same way as the patients, and then wonder why they do not comply with their treatment.

Examples of an external frame of reference include the following:

- 'Why don't you stop smoking?'
- 'You should lose weight.'
- 'You are getting too used to that bed.'
- 'You must get up for two hours today.'

These examples may seem a little extreme, but surely we have all heard them. When you try to get into your patient's frame of reference you will see things rather differently; for example:

- 'You did not understand what the doctor said and would like to have another word with him.'
- 'You are pleased about the results of the test.'
- 'You are worried about your children and are unsure whether your husband is coping.'
- 'You worry about your son's exams and feel helpless while being here.'
- 'You don't want to continue with the treatment but worry about your family's reactions.'

Do you see the difference? The examples show real understanding, they are also far less patronizing and will therefore foster a better relationship with people.

RISKS

Activity 8

It may be an idea to stop reading for a while and practise getting into people's frame of reference and see the world from their point of view, whenever you have a chance.

Next time you have a conversation with someone, for example, try to place yourself into her shoes and imagine what things look like from her point of view.

Discussion

Before we can communicate our appreciation of someone's point of view, we have to be receptive to that point of view and understand it. We have to come out of our shells, discard our professional distance and place ourselves alongside the patients (figuratively speaking, of course). This may sound easier than it is. It means that we must dismantle the elaborate system of defences we all have around us, and thus we may become more vulnerable. So there is an element of risk involved, but life is about risk-taking – if we never took any risks, none of us would even stir out of bed!

There is no-one as vulnerable as a patient. Patients take enormous risks by coming into hospital, or allowing us into their homes, and placing themselves at our mercy.

Risk-taking is essential for personal growth and development and, as with any development, the path may not always be smooth.

By placing ourselves alongside the patients we look after we may come face to face with issues, such as sexuality for example, we have not ourselves resolved. Or we may not have come to terms with our own mortality or with the death of our parents. So the path is far from smooth, but is exciting and can also be deeply satisfying.

Becoming open and available to people does not just mean giving; you will receive much in return, probably more than you expect. It is important, though, that you also remain open with your friends and colleagues and give them the opportunity to support you. You do not have to go it alone; after all, we are all in the same boat.

How do we show that we are willing to come alongside people? Well, first of all you have to be seen to be available. I am sure you have heard patients say, 'I did not like to bother the nurses, they work so hard.' OK, we do work hard, but who do we work hard for if it isn't the patients? If a patient thinks that a nurse is too busy to help her, that nurse must have communicated that to her. So what can be done to change that impression?

Activity 9

First of all, think how we communicate busy-ness or unavailability. You can do this activity either alone or in pairs.

Second, think how we can communicate that we are available and interested.

Third, go to a clinical area and, without taking part in any nursing care, simply observe what is going on. Can you see examples of the kind of 'busy-ness' we have been talking about? If so, how is it conveyed?

Discussion

It is likely that most of your answers concern non-verbal communication, the language of the body. Busy-ness and unavailability may be conveyed by rushing around, avoiding eye contact and remaining at the bottom of the bed.

Interest and availability, on the other hand, are signalled by slowing down and taking your time when you are with people. When you are talking with a patient, even if it is only for a short period, there is no reason why you cannot sit down. Also, if you remain standing while the patient is sitting or lying down, you may appear threatening as your physical position is unequal.

A relaxed, open posture is important, which means that you sit facing the other person without crossing your arms in self-defence. Other factors are a slight forward lean, which conveys interest, good eye contact, a friendly facial expression and head nods.

During a conversation it helps to ask open questions, which encourage people to say more. For example, instead of saying, 'Are you feeling all right?' you could say, 'How are you feeling?', or instead of, 'Does the prostatectomy operation worry you?', you could ask, 'How do you feel about your prostatectomy operation?'

There are many ways in which something can be said. Therefore, as we become more open and encourage people to talk to us, it is important that we are aware of the additional messages that accompany the spoken word.

Activity 10

List as many factors as you can think of which determine how you can say something.

The French have a good expression for it: 'C'est le ton qui fait la musique', which roughly translated means, 'It's not what you say, but the way that you say it'.

Factors which influence the way in which something is said include the following:

- volume (loud or barely audible);
- the pace of speech (fast or very slow);
- tone – a high voice, as when speaking to a baby, for example, or the deep boom of a command;
- variation, the stress on words or undifferentiated, monotonous speaking;
- clarity (easy or difficult to understand);
- accent (regional, foreign) – there is some research which suggests that people actually assign authority, intelligence and attractiveness to others depending on the accent with which they speak;
- disturbances – stammering, for example, may convey nervousness. Other paralinguistics include silences between words and rate or depth of breathing.

Activity 11

Whenever you have a chance, try and notice how people say things, and the effect this has.

Next time you see two people having a conversation, listen to what they are saying and how they are saying it. Notice what is really going on.

BODY LANGUAGE

We hear a lot about body language these days, but what is it? Well it involves quite a list. Here are some of the factors which may be involved:

- eye contact and looking;
- smiling, laughing;
- facial expression;
- gesture;
- hand movements, fidgeting;
- leg movements, bouncing, crossing and uncrossing legs;
- position of body, relaxed, tense;
- leaning forward or leaning back;
- orientation, towards or away from the speaker;

- touch, presence or absence, appropriateness;
- distance between people, usually greater between men than between women;
- clothes, hair style, hair colour (natural?);
- breathing;
- blushing.

Good observation of body language is an extremely important nursing skill. Often patients do not say outright how they feel, that they are worried or in pain, because they are afraid of being thought difficult or a nuisance. It is therefore essential that nurses become attuned to picking up people's body signals.

Activity 12

This activity is designed to practise listening to people's body language. It is a bit like the children's game 'Simon Says'. Talk to a partner for two or three minutes. While you are talking, your partner tries to copy your body languge. After two minutes your partner tells you what she thought your body was saying. Was she right?

Reverse the roles. You can play this as often as you like. Practising it with different people will give you even more insight.

Activity 13

Next time you are out with someone, having coffee at a restaurant, for example, see if you can both observe the same person, without it becoming obvious, for a few moments. Discuss how you interpreted the other person's body language and see whether you are in agreement.

THINGS THAT GET IN THE WAY

As these activities may have shown, it is not always easy to interpret accurately someone else's communication. This is because in any communication there is a wealth of potential information to be received. In everyday life only a small fraction of that information is attended to, that is, selective attention is employed. This is done because too much information might interfere with the job in hand, and therefore one concentrates on what seems relevant at the time. In addition, all our perceptions are passed through a kind of filter, which is very personal to us. Such a filter is developed through our previous experiences of people and situations as well as our interests. Thus, if Mrs Jones is talking to Mrs Davies, who is a policewoman, her perception of her will be influenced by Mrs Jones' previous experience of policewomen in general. As a result, Mrs Jones may fail to listen accurately to Mrs Davies and receive a different message to the one which has actually been sent.

Selective attention and filtering are the two major reasons why communications are often unsatisfactory, as no-one really listens accurately. Therefore, as the quote by Lao Tse (page 117) illustrates, in order to listen accurately, we have to begin with ourselves. We have to listen to ourselves and become aware of what goes on within ourselves. In order to do this we need a quality of stillness and of silence. This may not be easy because modern men and women are forever rushing around, constantly hungry for impressions and entertainment, yet filtering out much of what is available. Activity 6 on page 118 is one method to develop such 'inner listening', meditation is another.

As any communication is a two-way process, it follows that factors involving the talker can also influence the accuracy of one's understanding.

Activity 14

Think of factors which may interfere with your listening, factors to do with the person who is doing the talking. What kind of things about a person could distract your attention away from what they are saying to you? Try to think of real people and actual situations.

Jot down your ideas and discuss them with a partner.

Discussion

You may have included factors such as differences between you and the other person's age, sex, culture or socio-economic background.

Other factors include physical problems, such as with speech, for example, following a stroke, or breathlessness. Tiredness, anxiety, shyness or confusion may also inhibit one's understanding.

Activity 15

With a partner, take turns in talking and listening for a few minutes. As well as listening to your partner, try to listen to what goes on inside yourself. You could talk about the last holiday you had, or the one you are planning to take this year. (Five minutes each).

Discuss what kind of things you noticed about yourself.

Discussion

There are many things that can interfere with listening to people. They may be physical aspects, such as tiredness, headache, hearing or vision problems. Other factors may include not having enough time, being worried or preoccupied or thinking about what you are going to say next.

It is not only internal things which may distract you; outside factors also play a part, such as noise or the presence of many other people.

As nursing is a caring profession, we often feel that we have to do something when faced with a patient's distress, which may get in the way of accurate listening. We feel that we have to reassure, which may not be what the patient wants or needs; it may also be dishonest.

SHOWING THAT YOU UNDERSTAND

When you are talking to someone who is interested and under-standing, you are encouraged to go on talking. But how do you know that the other person is interested and understanding? What messages do they send which make you want to go on talking?

Messages that show interest include non-verbal signals such as looking, nodding, smiling and appropriate facial expressions in response to what is being said. It would be disconcerting, for example, if one continued to smile on being told something rather sad.

One can show interest verbally, too, by saying things such as: 'Go on; really?' and, 'then? Hmm, hmm,' and so on.

It is a good experience to be really listened to, which makes people feel valued. However, it is very important that the verbal and non-verbal messages agree with each other, in other words, your non-verbal behaviour must be congruent with what you are saying. If one's non-verbal behaviour does not agree with what is being said – for example, if we say we are glad but look bored – this will be experienced as insincerity and will discourage people from talking further.

Activity 16

With a partner, take turns at talking and listening. When listening, give verbal signs of encouragement, but let your non-verbal behaviour be unmatching. For example, say, 'Really, go on', but do not look at your partner. You will probably be able to think of many more ways in which your verbal and non-verbal behaviour can be made to disagree.

Discuss how that felt. Did you go on talking? Apart from not matching what you are saying, it is also possible to give discouraging non-verbal messages. Think of what kind of non-verbal behaviour you may find discouraging.

Discussion

Nurses and doctors are particularly good at discouraging body language. Standing at a distance, for example, at the bottom of the bed, standing while the patient is in bed, clutching notes – these are all things we do every day. But even if you are sitting and talking with someone it is still possible to put people off; fidgeting, bouncing a leg up and down, an exaggerated laid-back position, sitting turned away from someone, not really looking at the person or looking blank, these are all examples.

Usually discouraging behaviour is experienced as a put-down. Basically, one is being told, 'OK, I'm here because I have to be, but I'm not interested in you or what you are saying', or 'I'm too polite to say, but what you are saying is rubbish.'

Another way in which we put people down without meaning to is by inappropriately reassuring people. We often do this by saying things like, 'Don't worry, you'll be all right', when it is very likely that the person will not be all right and has every reason to worry.

Think of ways in which people tend to reassure us and we reassure others. Examples include saying:

- 'You'll be all right';
- 'You'll grow out of it';
- 'Cheer up, it may never happen';
- 'Never mind, you've still got ...';
- 'Never mind, you're young enough to have another baby.'

Other inappropriate ways in which we tend to reassure people include taking the opportunity to start talking about ourselves;

- 'I know just how you feel, when I ... ';
- 'That's just what happened to me when ... ';
- 'I can understand that; when I ... '

Activity 17

With a partner, take turns to tell each other about a problem (two minutes each). The listener replies with one or more of the above expressions.

How did that feel?

Discussion

Most people experience these types of answers as a put-down, or as a message to shut up and stop whining. Not only is the message given unhelpful, it may also be untrue. It may not be all right. Or , even if it will be all right, you do not know that, unless you have second sight.

Nurses are also likely to be patronizing or too ready with advice, without giving people a chance to come to their own solution.

Activity 18

You need a partner. One of you is a compulsive smoker; you are in hospital for the third time this year with a chest infection, but take every opportunity to sneak to the toilet for a crafty fag. The other person is the nurse in her role of health educator; she is a non-smoker and strongly disapproves of patients who endanger their health by smoking. (Eight to ten minutes).

Afterwards discuss how the conversation felt for each of you. Was the nurse helpful? Did she persuade you to stop smoking? Or are you so upset that you will just have to have a cigarette to calm you down? What would have been helpful?

Discussion

It may be helpful to look out for examples of what has been discussed in this last section, both at work and in your private life. Once you become aware of how we behave it is fascinating to see just how rich a repertoire of non-verbal as well as verbal behaviour we all have.

WHAT DO I SAY?

Until now we have discussed how you can let a person know that you are interested in what they are saying. Ways of doing this include encouraging non-verbal messages as well as verbal responses (such as 'hmm, hmm', 'go on', 'really?' and so on). We also talked about the undesirability of inappropriate reassurance or advice. In addition, we have concentrated on what not to do. You may now wonder if there is anything you can do or say that is going to be helpful.

Do not worry. If you are really interested and concerned about the other person and do your best to see things from their point of view, it is likely that you communicate this without realizing it. You probably are, as Barrett-Lennard calls it, 'responding with empathy'.

There are various ways in which you can demonstrate your understanding. Two such methods are paraphrasing and reflection.

Paraphrasing

Paraphrasing basically restates what someone says, for example:

Patient   *'I am worried about my business – there is no-one to take care of it while I'm in here.'*

Nurse   *'You are worried about being in here when there is no-one to take care of your business.'*

or

Patient   *'The doctor says I can go home, but I'm not sure I can cope.'*

Nurse   *'You feel unsure whether you can cope, even though the doctor says you can go home.'*

or

Patient	*'Since my husband died last year I have not really managed to get out much as we always used to do everything together.'*
Nurse	*'You feel unsure about going out alone as you are not used to doing things by yourself.'*

or

Patient	*'I do not think the treatment is doing anything as I feel worse now than before I came in.'*
Nurse	*'You are worried that you do not seem to be getting any better and wonder if you are having the right treatment.'*

Paraphrasing may seem artificial at first, but it is actually quite encouraging. It demonstrates that you are listening and have understood what has been said. People then feel free to go on and supply further information. For example, the patient in the first example may go on to say 'Yes, you see I am self-employed and have no other source of income ...'

Activity 19

With a partner, take turns in attempting paraphrasing. The more you do it, the easier it will become. You could talk about what you plan to do on your next day off, or what you did on the last free day you had.

Discuss how it felt afterwards (20 minutes).

Reflection

Reflection is like paraphrasing, but instead of relating the actual content of what someone is saying, one reflects the underlying feeling.

Activity 20

Again, take turns at talking and listening with your partner. You could talk about people in the public eye and what you think about them, for example. When you have the role of the listener, practise reflecting the underlying feeling of each other's statements, rather than the actual content (5 minutes each).

Discussion

It is not easy, is it? How did it feel? Reflection is a little bit more difficult than paraphrasing as there is always the possibility of making an error. If you are unsure, you could say, after your response, 'Is that right?', or 'Have I understood that correctly?', to give the other person a chance to correct you.

If you have a good relationship with someone and they realize that you are genuine in your interest, it is likely that they will correct you of their own accord, even without you asking. They may say, 'Well, no, not quite, what I mean is . . .'. A useful ploy is to start your reflection with, 'You feel . . .', which will make it easier to say things from the other person's point of view.

Some examples are as follows:

Patient	*'I do not think the operation was worth it. The cancer may have gone, but now that I have only got one breast left, who is going to look at me?'*
Nurse	*'You are feeling less attractive now because of the loss of your breast, which is making you feel depressed and worried that you may never find a man who will love you and accept you as you are.'*

or

Student	*'I am not happy on the ward, the trained staff are always picking on me and I do not think that I am learning anything.'*
Teacher	*'You feel angry and unhappy because the ward staff are not treating you as part of the team.'*

or

Ward sister	*'I am fed up trying to do the off duty. We are so short staffed that I just cannot give the girls the time off they want.'*
Senior sister	*'You feel frustrated because you do not have sufficient staff on the ward. This makes it difficult for you to give staff the off duty they want and they are not happy about this.'*

Of course, in reflection you still take all the non-verbal communications into account as well, as they will probably give additional clues regarding the underlying feeling of what is being said.

CONCLUSION

Listening is the most important part of helping and counselling and is, initially in any case, often all that is required. You may find that patients start saying to you, 'You are the first person who has really listened to me.' This may or may not be true, you may not be the first person who has listened, but you may be the first person who has demonstrated to that patient that she is listening.

Once you really listen to people you will be far less likely to judge and label, as you will understand why they behave the way they do. Many of the problems which occur within hospitals between the various groups, such as nurses and patients/relatives, doctors and nurses, nurses and nurses, are due to a lack of communication – no-one is really listening.

There is a well-known saying, 'If you want to change the world, start with yourself'. You may well find that your listening skills rub off on other people, and that they start to listen, too, and become appreciative of your point of view.

Of course, there is much more to communication, listening and counselling. Learning about it is really a life-long process. Ideally, we never stop learning and developing; that is what is so exciting.

Chapter 7 will apply the listening and counselling skills discussed to the specific area of sexuality as affected by illness.

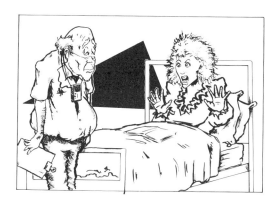

REFERENCES

Barrett-Lennard, G.T. (1981) The empathy cycle: refinement of a nuclear concept. *Journal of Counselling Psychology*, **28**, 91–100.

Bundy, C. (1989) Cardiac disorders, in *Health Psychology; Processes and Applications* (ed. A. Broome), Chapman & Hall, London.

Burnard, P. (1987) Developing skills as a group facilitator. *The Professional Nurse*, October, **3**(1), 19–22.

Gruen, W. (1975) Effects of brief psychotherapy during the hospitalization period on the recovery process in heart attacks. *Journal of Consulting and Clinical Psychology*, **43**, 223–32.

Matthews, B.P. (1962) Measurement of psychological aspects of the nurse–patient relationship. *Nursing Research*, **11**(3), 154–62.

Mazzuca, S. (1982) Does patient education in chronic disease have therapeutic value? *Journal of Chronic Disease*, **35**, 521–9.
Nurse, G. (1980) Counselling and helping skills: how can they be learned? 1 and 2.*Nursing Times*, **1**, 15.
Royal College of Nursing (1978) *Counselling in Nursing*. The report of a working party held under the auspices of the RCN Institute of Advanced Nursing Education, RCN, London.
Schlesinger, H., Mumford, E., Glass, G. *et al*. (1983) Mental health treatment and medical care. *American Journal of Public Health*, **73**, 422–9.
Truax, C.B. and Miller (1971) Perceived therapeutic conditions offered by contrasting occupations. Unpublished manuscript.

FURTHER READING

Bond, M. (1986) *Stress and Self-Awareness: A Guide for Nurses*, Heinemann, London.
Burnard, P. (1990) *Learning Human Skills. A Guide for Nurses*, Heinemann, London.
Nelson-Jones, R. (1988) *Practical Counselling and Helping Skills*, 2nd edn, Cassell, London.
Rogers, C.R. (1951) *Client-Centered Therapy*, Constable, London.

Sexuality and illness

LEARNING OBJECTIVES

After reading this chapter you should be able to:

1. outline how nurses may assess sexuality and actual or potential problems;
2. discuss how sexuality may be affected by illness in general;
3. discuss specific problems caused by a number of conditions and identify helping strategies.

ASSESSMENT

Some models of nursing, such as that of Roper, Logan and Tierney (1980), explicitly state sexuality as a relevant factor to be assessed. However, even if they do not explicitly mention sexuality, most models, to a greater or lesser extent, take a holistic point of view, and therefore sexuality is included implicitly. But what is there to be assessed and how does one go about it? Going up to a patient and saying 'How about your sexuality, then, Mr Jones – any problems?' is likely to meet with a frosty reception.

Activity 1

First, jot down the various aspects of sexuality which you think are relevant when assessing a patient and, second, think of ways in which you would go about this.

Discussion

As Chapter 3, on sexuality and ethics, describes, nurses often concentrate on what a patient looks like, whether they like to use toiletries and occasionally they may make reference to the fact that the patient is married. But that is usually as far as it goes. In order to do a proper assessment, however, and to identify actual and potential problems, nurses need to do more than that. First, we need to have an idea of how the particular condition a patient has (as well as its treatment) can affect a person's sexuality. Second, we need to know to what extent this is the case for the actual patient we are assessing. As every patient is an individual, illness will affect them in different ways, and one can never assume anything. The kind of factors which are relevant to a person's sexuality are many, and include their upbringing, the way they think, feel and behave, their environment, culture, religion and society, the patient's personal circumstances and how he or she feels about them, and physical aspects and how they are affected by the illness.

Figure 7.1 sets out how a person's experience in the 'here and now' is influenced by all of these aspects.

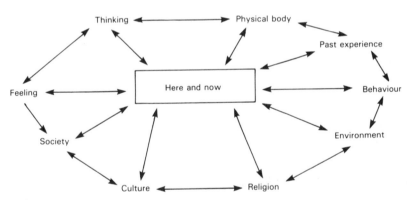

Figure 7.1 The 'here and now', and how it is influenced.

Activity 2

Before going any further, take each category from Figure 7.1 and list all the aspects which you think may be relevant. Better still, have a brainstorm with a few others. Experience, for example, might include gender, sexual orientation, actual circumstances at present, whether single, married or in a relationship, past relationships, and so on.

Discussion

The following lists are not exclusive; it is quite possible that you came up with additional factors. However, taken together, it does provide a framework to bear in mind when assessing someone. It is not suggested that you ask a patient questions on each factor – that would seem too much like an interrogation as well as possibly an infringement of privacy. It is useful though to bear in mind the general framework, in the same way that you would probably bear in mind the social, emotional, psychological and physical aspects of each activity of living when assessing a patient according to the Roper, Logan and Tierney (1980) model, for example.

Body

- State of health normally, and current state of ill health.
- Body image normally and how affected by current illness.
- Physical effects of ill health.
- Physical effects of treatment or surgery.
- Side-effects of drugs.

Behaviour

- Sexual behaviour normally when healthy.
- How affected by illness and treatment.
- Desired sexual functioning at present.

Society

- Linked to culture.
- Occupation, class – attitudes to sexuality.
- Social mores adhered to.

Culture

- Non-British, if so, which culture plus all that entails?
- If British, which part?

Religion

- Which religion?
- Views held by the individual, as even within a religion they may vary? Some Roman Catholics, for example, will practise birth control, although officially artificial methods are against the teaching of the Roman Catholic church.

Thinking

- Beliefs about sexuality in general.
- Beliefs about self and sexuality.
- Beliefs about the way in which illness and treatment has affected sexuality or could possibly do so in the future.

Feeling

- Linked to body image and self-esteem.
- How comfortable with own sexuality?
- How comfortable with their social role of breadwinner, housewife, career woman, and so on?
- How happy with normal level of functioning?
- Feelings about how the illness and treatment has affected sexuality.
- Feelings about any relationships the patient has.

Of course, none of the above categories are discrete, they are all interlinked and interdependent. The state of physical well-being, for example, will affect how people feel about themselves and is likely to influence their body image and self-esteem as well as their sexual relationships.

So, when assessing a patient on sexuality it is important to bear all these factors in mind, and to establish the normal state of affairs and how the illness has altered things. Having established how the various aspects of sexuality have been affected by the illness, it should be possible to ascertain which actually present a problem to the patient. Some effects may be transient and resolve once the condition of the patient improves. Others, however, may be longer term or even permanent. As with all problem identification, it should be a problem as far as the patient is concerned, and not the nurse. It is possible, for example, that the nurse has identified loss of hair by chemotherapy as being a problem for a man, whereas he may not be particularly concerned about that.

Active listening skills, as discussed in Chapter 6, are very useful in obtaining the information needed to make an assessment. Much of the information will probably be discovered in caring for the patient as part of normal conversation. The following types of open questions may be useful to find out more.

- 'How has your illness affected the way you feel about yourself?'
- 'Sometimes people with your condition worry whether it is OK to have sexual relations; is there anything you would like to ask me?'
- 'People sometimes worry about the fact that they do not seem to have much interest in sex; how about you?'

SEXUALITY

Picture yourself with a streaming cold. You cannot stop sneezing, your throat hurts, your eyes water and you have a major headache. Do you feel attractive? Sexy? In the mood? What about your body image? Chances are that you are slopping around the house in old pyjamas or tracksuit clutching a hot water bottle and a large box of tissues. In other words, unless you are a very unusual being, you feel singularly awful and unattractive and probably just want to be left alone or tucked up in bed, with someone refreshing the hot water bottle from time to time and bringing you cold remedies and light refreshments. Being sexy is very likely to be the last thing on your mind.

While carrying out the research for this chapter, one man made the following comment:

> *Why do you need to write a book about sexuality and illness? It's pretty obvious, isn't it? When you are ill you don't feel like it and there is nothing you can do about it. Either you fancy it or you don't. Anyway, what has it got to do with nurses? What can they do about it?*

It is certainly true that during the acute stage of any infection, being sexy is not a primary concern for most people. However, even so people can be helped to feel better about themselves and in themselves by having shower or bath, putting on attractive, freshly laundered clothes or sleepwear, and having a clean bed to step into with freshly changed bed linen. As was seen in Chapters 4 and 5, on how men and women see the world, sexuality means much more to people than simply the sex act. It is integral to how we feel as a man or a woman, how we feel about our bodies as well as about ourselves as people, and how we relate to people in general. In other words, our sexuality infuses everything we do every moment of the day; it is very much part of us and cannot be separated out. Whether or not we are sexually active is another matter. It is possible for people to feel very desirable and generally satisfied with themselves, and yet because of choice or circumstance, they do not have an active sex life. Also, it is not something that is static; people can go through months or even years of having a low libido, followed by a period of high activity.

Activity 3

Why should this be so? Why does people's libido vary? What reasons can you think of?

Discussion

The obvious reason for an altered libido is acute illness. When people are busy feeling really ill, their libido is probably practically non-existent for a while. However, there are a myriad of other causes; any change in circumstance, whether physical, emotional or social, may have an effect. Precisely because sexuality is so much a part of what and who we are, it is also easily affected by whatever is going on in our lives. Stress, overwork and tiredness are common reasons for people to lose interest in sex. A woman who is holding down a part-time job to help make ends meet as well as looking after a young family and an elderly, dependent father, has probably very little energy left for anything else. Also, a busy executive, who goes from meeting to meeting, meets deadline after deadline and is never far away from the computer terminal, fax machine and carphone, may have so much on his mind that there is little room for anything else.

However, circumstances which appear to be similar on the surface may affect people in different ways. The harassed woman in the above example might equally well regard getting into bed with her husband as an ideal way to unwind and really enjoy making love with him and spending time on something they both enjoy. The stressed executive may actually thrive on stress and find it enhances his interest in sex. He may well have an active sex life with his wife as well as a rampant affair with a girl from the typing pool. Who knows? People are different, that is the important thing to bear in mind, and we should never assume that we know how events affect them.

In making themselves available to patients regarding sexuality and related problems, therefore, nurses should use the active listening skills discussed in Chapter 6. It is important to bear in mind that real listening, where people feel that they are being heard and understood, is not just a trick or skill, but a 'way of being' (Rogers, 1980). We must really want to listen, mean it, be genuine, have an entirely open mind and, above all, be non-judgemental. No matter what people tell us, we should take care not to judge or label them as that will get in the way of the helping process. As soon as we find ourselves judging people, or labelling a 75-year-old with an interest in sex as 'a dirty old man', for example, we are not available for the patient. We have placed ourselves separate from him, not alongside him.

It is possible that on occasion someone may tell you something that they think, do or have done of which you disapprove or with which you disagree. That is only natural, we are all different and have varying preferences and desires. However, when that occurs it is important to distinguish the view or act from the person. As Rogers (1980) says, it is perfectly possible to disagree with something someone has done while still prizing them as a person. In other words, we should not condemn people for just one particular aspect or deed. In any case, we all do things and have done things of which we are not all that proud, whether in relation to sexuality or anything else. Being non-judgemental is an important issue for nursing as judging leads to label-ing which, as Stockwell (1972) first showed, has real implications for the actual nursing care people receive.

Activity 4

Have you ever been at the receiving end of people judging or labelling you? Has anyone ever said to you something like, 'I would have thought that you . . . ' or, 'You are a typical . . . aren't you?' and been way off the mark? How did that make you feel? If you are lucky enough not to have been in this position, find a few other people and discuss it. Alternatively, you could purposely describe each other in unexpected ways and see how that feels.

Scenario

Sue, a teacher, was having a discussion with Tim and a few other colleagues about what they did in their spare time, and happened to say that it was not necessarily true that women did not enjoy having a pint or watching football. Tim turned to her and said: 'You are turning into a staunch feminist, aren't you, Sue?' Sue was taken aback. Whereas she certainly regarded herself as a fairly liberated woman, she was aware that for many people the term 'feminist' has very negative connotations. She therefore asked Tim what, in his opinion, a feminist was. Tim said:'Oh, they are anti-men and tend to be very aggressive. I was thrown out of a shop once because it was run by women and men were not supposed to be there.'

Sue failed to see what Tim's rather idiosyncratic view of feminists had do with her (or indeed with most feminists), nor how her remark, which was meant as a statement of fact, could be construed as proof of her being that kind of woman. Sue liked men, she knew that men usually found her attractive and was, in fact, rarely without a boyfriend for long. Tim's image of her as an angry, aggressive man-hating creature was therefore com-pletely alien to her and actually really upset her. 'If one person can see me so differently,' she thought, 'how many other people see me like that as well?'

Tim, realizing that she was upset, asked her what was the matter and she told him. Now it was his turn to be taken aback. Seeing Sue in the way he did, vulnerability or being upset was somehow not something he thought she was prone to. This led to a discussion, after which they realized that, in fact, Tim's view of Sue had more to do with him than with her. In other words, he saw Sue through the glasses of his own opinions, prejudices and previous experiences, not as she really was.

Discussion

Being judged is not always hurtful, it can also be flattering. It may depend on the circumstances. What seems appropriate in one situation may not be so in another. The person doing the judging is also significant; it is more hurtful to be misjudged by someone whom we know fairly well, or someone we care about, than someone who we do not particularly like anyway or who is only a very casual acquaintance. Patients in hospital are in a vulnerable position, they place themselves in our care, and may be at a low emotional ebb. Therefore, they have the right to expect nurses to 'take care'. Being in the position of a nurse and having people place their trust in you is actually a great privilege. It is therefore important to get it right, to try and really 'see and hear' people as they are, not as we think they appear or might be.

Activity 5

Before going on, complete the following statements:

- If I were ill I would worry about . . .
- If I were ill my problems would be . . .
- If I were ill I would want nurses to . . .

Discussion

The same three statements were completed by 31 qualified nurses and third-year nursing students. All were female and aged between 20 and 50, with a mean age of 31. Their responses were as follows:

If I were ill I would worry about . . .

Responses to this statement were very varied, but tended to fall into five categories: appearance, relationships, illness-related, social and practical factors.

(a) Appearance
Ten people were concerned with their appearance, which included wanting to be clean and tidy, wanting to have their hair washed and styled in the usual way, preventing body odour and cleaning teeth.

(b) Relationships
This included being unable to fulfil the normal role of wife, mother and housekeeper; six people were concerned with this.

The effect on the partner and family is also mentioned by six people, whereas one person said she would worry about her relationship with her partner, and two people mentioned they would worry about not being able to make love.

(c) Illness-related
This included concerns with diagnosis, outcome and recovery, and was mentioned by eight people. Six people were concerned with dying, and one person with sexually transmitted disease.

(d) Social
Six people said they would worry about their job, and three people would worry about financial problems.

(e) Practical factors
This included pain (one person), dignity (two people) and hospital admission (four people).

Two people said they would worry about it being known that she was a nurse and being expected to know everything.

If I were ill my problems would be ...

Nine people's problems would be due to being away from the family and worrying about who would look after the children. Not being able to care for themselves and being helpless was seen as a problem by six people. Eleven people mentioned that they would have job-related and financial problems.

Eighteen people mentioned a variety of problems which were illness-related. They included worry, fear, anxiety and depression (eight people), loss of dignity (two people), pain and nausea (two people) and coping problems (two people), whereas four people saw their main problem as getting well again.

If I were ill I would want nurses to . . .

The kind of things people wanted nurses to do fell into two main categories; (1) appearance and hygiene, and (2) psychological and emotional care.

(a) Appearance and hygiene
Nine people were concerned with their appearance and hygiene; particular concerns appeared to be the care of hair and teeth and the prevention of body odour. A few people were very detailed in how they would like to be looked after.

(b) Psychological and emotional care
Twenty-one people's answers came under this category. They were very varied and included the following: treat me as a person and not as an illness or a nurse, listen, advise, reassure, give me time to voice fears, leave me alone to have a cry, treat me with respect and dignity, respect my privacy, appreciate my sexuality, and be supportive, sympathetic, empathetic and caring.

Three people wanted to be left alone as much as possible, with nurses doing the minimum. One person, however, summed it all up by saying, 'I would want nurses to care about me'.

This last sentence is actually very poignant, as nurses do a great deal of caring 'for', but to what extent do they always care 'about' a patient? Can we as nurses honestly say that we always care equally about each and every patient? Yet, if we are honest, is that not what we would want for ourselves? In a way, if we really care about a patient, we cannot but give good care, which includes a wide variety of issues, as shown above. If we treat people as individuals and care **about** as well as **for** them holistically, then sexuality and how it is affected by illness cannot be left out.

ILLNESS

The expression of sexuality, whether by appearance, behaviour or sexual relations, is usually restored once the patient gets better. Some conditions, however, such as myocardial infarction, diabetes, arthritis or chronic respiratory disease, have a more lasting effect. In addition, if people are having problems with their relationship, then sooner or later it will also have effects on their sex life. In such a situation the additional burden posed by illness – especially if the illness or the treatment causes problems with sexuality – may be in danger of becoming the 'last straw' for the relationship. Things will be made very much worse if the people concerned do not know that the sexual problems are related to the disease.

Problems

So what kind of problems may be caused by illness? Ilness-related problems with sexuality are not isolated, they are very much interwoven with everything else that is going on in someone's life. Ill health in itself has psychological and emotional repercussions, apart from the obvious physical problems. Ill health is often associated with mental as well as physical fatigue. Drugs may cause additional problems. The effects of traumatic events, such as bereavement, should not be underestimated. Bereavement has a profound effect on people's physical and emotional well-being, and it is not uncommon for people to suffer ill health following a bereavement. Emotional pain, whether caused by a bereavement or by other upsetting events, may manifest itself physically. People may experience tiredness, have headaches, backache or other aches and pain. Women's menstrual cycles may be disrupted, and periods may become irregular or unusually prolonged, or there may be vaginal discharge. Both sexes may experience a decrease in libido, which is a reflection of their reduced well-being generally. Unless these processes are understood, it is likely that if sexual problems occur they will affect a relationship. Conversely, if the relationship itself is problematic then this will eventually manifest itself in sexual problems.

Activity 6

What effects in general do you think illness and treatment, whether by surgery or by drugs, may have on sexuality?

Discussion

The effects of illness and treatment may be emotional as well as physical. Depending on the condition, physical problems may include pain, a reduction in strength and mobility, paralysis, fatigue, incontinence or breathlessness. The person may have a catheter or stoma. All these physical effects will influence how the person is feeling emotionally as well as sexually.

Emotional effects include embarrassment, particularly if there is a change in how the body looks or feels, and loss of self-esteem or a poor body image, causing people to feel sexually unattractive or disgusted with themselves. If the condition is irreversible, or if there has been mutilating surgery, the person may be grieving for the loss of a healthy body. If the person is in a relationship both partners may be grieving, as both will be affected. Frequently people experience anxiety about the effects of sexual activity on the medical condition. In the case of a person with cancer, for example, the partner may also feel guilty about seeking sexual pleasure from a person who is very ill.

In the case of long-term ill health, people may feel unhappy about the change in their social role; they may have had to give up work, or reduce their activity in the home, for example. An overall result of the various emotional problems may be depression, which may manifest itself in a lack of energy, insomnia or disturbances in appetite. Sexual problems include reduced libido, impotence or frigidity and an inability to reach orgasm.

AGE

Somehow our culture celebrates the young, but does not value the older members of society. As regards sexuality, the young get the message that 'everybody is doing it all the time' whereas older people are often regarded as asexual. Although this is certainly not the case and, indeed, many people in their 70s and beyond enjoy a fulfilling sex life, many older people are affected by these societal messages. In addition, ill health and its related problems are more common among the elderly, who may also worry and grieve about the loss of their youth, looks and vitality. Sometimes people are too quick to see any problems as inevitable: 'What can you expect at my age?' is a commonly heard phrase. The answer is 'you can expect a great deal'. There is no reason why age alone should be a hindrance to people's sexual expression. Indeed, a survey by the Association of Retired Persons, reported in *The Guardian* (1990), found that the majority of people over 60 were enjoying sex as much as earlier in their lives (75% of men and 72% of women).

It is sometimes thought that women's interest in sex declines after the menopause. This is an interesting issue as until the turn of the century, the average life expectancy was only 48. Sexuality past the age of childbearing was therefore not an issue that was in people's awareness, which may account for the assumption 'no sex please, I'm past the menopause'. It appears that the menopause itself is not significant with regard to a woman's interest in sex. For some women it is even increased as she no longer has to worry about getting pregnant. For those women where interest does decline, there is a direct relation with the period prior to the menopause. In other words, women who have never been particularly interested are likely to be even less interested in their later years. For most women, however, the menopause itself does not have a significant impact on the level of their sexual activity and enjoyment.

In fact, for women as well as men, it appears that the quality of people's sex lives very much depends on the level of sexual activity enjoyed for the earlier part of their lives, and whether this level has been maintained (Masters and Johnson, 1966). As with all age-related changes, maintenance of activity is vitally important. Sometimes, however, an elderly person may be temporarily without a partner, possibly because of divorce, illness or bereavement, but fully intends to start another relationship if the opportunity presents itself. For such a person, whether male or female, masturbation is an effective way to keep the sexual organs active as well as offering some physical relief.

When today's elderly population were in their formative years, sex was very much a taboo subject and they were not brought up to discuss sexual matters. Consequently, in contrast with younger age groups, many old people today would not discuss sexual problems with even very close friends (*The Guardian*, 1990). Therefore some elderly people may turn to nurses (or doctors) for advice on sexual matters as they see nurses as professional people who do not get embarrassed and may be able to help. Others, however, may be more reluctant and subtly hint at problems. This is where skilled listening is so important, as failure to respond to the hints may mean that the patient will not raise the issue again.

Fred and Ethel

Fred and Ethel had been married for 48 years and were looking forward to celebrating their diamond wedding anniversary in two years' time. Although they had had their ups and downs, theirs was basically a good marriage. While their five children were young, things were a little turbulent at times, but since they had left home Fred and Ethel found that, in a way, they had got to know and appreciate each other all over again. Ethel had never worked outside the home and had therefore to get used to Fred being around so much after he retired from his job as a maintenance worker on the railways.

Neither had received much sex education in their youth, and in fact Ethel had been brought up to believe that it was all rather sordid and dirty. Like many women at that time, Ethel was still a virgin when she married Fred, aged 18, and was not expecting anything particularly pleasurable from sexual relations. Fred was a few years older, had travelled a bit and had gained some experience sexually. So Ethel was delighted to discover that sex with Fred was wonderful. 'I'm so lucky', she said. 'I know that many women my age have never really enjoyed sex, and are only too happy to give it up as soon as they can get away with it. They don't know what they are missing.' Now aged 76 and

80, Ethel and Fred still enjoy an active sex life. They are happy to be alive, and to still have each other's company.

'There was a period though', said Fred, 'when our children thought it rather distasteful that we were still having sexual relations. The subject came up one day through one of the grandchildren asking questions, and I naturally got involved in the conversation. However, we have talked it through and the children are now actually delighted and say that they are now less worried about getting old as they can see how much we are still enjoying life and each other.'

Discussion

Fred and Ethel are lucky. Whatever problems they encountered regarding their sexuality, they were able to discuss it together and use commonsense methods to overcome them. It would not be true to say that age does not change how people look, feel and behave, we all know otherwise. However, many of the problems that we associate with old age are not actually part of the normal ageing process but due to a specific illness. Although conditions such as stroke, parkinsonism or arthritis can occur at any age, it is true that there is a higher incidence of these and other illnesses in older people. It is important to remember, though, that these conditions are definitely not part of the normal ageing process and many people stay well and healthy.

Regarding sexuality, there are a number of changes associated with the ageing process. For men as well as women over the age of 60, the speed with which they become aroused tends to slow down. For both sexes the sex organs become less sensitive, that is, the penis in men, and the vulva and vagina, and occasionally the breasts, in women. Also, the erection angle of the penis is reduced, there is less ejaculate fluid and it takes longer to ejaculate and recover before another erection can take place. These changes can actually be beneficial, as the delay may mean enhanced pleasure for both partners.

For some women, sex may become uncomfortable or even painful, due to the fact that post menopausal hormonal changes cause the vaginal mucosa to become thinner, more fragile and less moist. This is what Ethel experienced, but she found that using a water-based lubricant overcame the problem quite effectively. She found out that oils or vaseline, although equally effective, were not a good idea as they may increase the risk of infection to which elderly women are more prone. Ethel also found that her bladder tended to get irritated during intercourse, but she coped with this by urinating beforehand. There may also be a reduction in the number of orgasms a woman experiences, although as with all these age-related changes, there is great individual variation. Regular sexual activity is important in the maintenance and healthy functioning of the sexual organs, and for women regular actual contact with a penis helps maintain the integrity of the vagina.

An important reason why some elderly people's sex lives become less satisfactory is due to psychological and social factors, rather than physical causes. Some couples may simply have fallen out of love, or be bored with each other, and only stay together out of habit. Not only are couples in this position less likely to have an active sex life, they are probably also less close generally. So they are less likely to kiss and cuddle or put their arms around each other. As discussed previously, there is more to sexuality than the sex act. Physical contact, not necessarily related to sexual relations, is actually an important part of being human and helps to maintain a feeling of well-being.

Ethel and Fred hugged and cuddled a great deal, which seemed a natural expression of their affection for each other. 'It does not matter that we do not necessarily have an orgasm every time we make love,' said Fred. 'We get a lot of enjoyment out of just being close and appreciating each other.'

ARTHRITIS

Chronic diseases such as arthritis tend to be characterized by periods of exacerbation and remission as well as by phases of relative stability. As the disease is progressive, people can at times get really depressed, especially during a phase when the disease flares up. They may feel really tired, have many aches and pains and be generally fed up with everything, wondering what the point is of carrying on. Once in a period of remission, however, people often feel wonderful and enjoy the respite, hoping that it will last a long time.

Susan

Susan is a 52-year-old married woman, whose children are grown up. Over the past three years Susan has developed arthritis, which started in her hands and then gradually spread to other parts of her body. Until a few months ago, Susan and her husband had a reasonably active sex life, but due to pain and discomfort, intercourse became less and less frequent until about a month ago when it stopped altogether.

In a way, Susan feels relieved as the pain during intercourse became too much, but she also feels bad as she loves George and feels they are too young to give up on a normal relationship. Also she feels it is unfair on George.

During a visit to her GP for an evaluation of her drug regime, she had a chat with Angie, the practice nurse. As she had become a regular visitor to the surgery, Angie had got to know Susan and asked her how she was getting on. 'Oh, all right I suppose', said Susan, 'but, you know, I suppose it is downhill from now on, really, isn't it?' Angie sensed that something was the matter and felt that Susan was dropping a subtle hint, whether she realized it or not. 'Come and sit down for a few minutes,' she said. 'I haven't got anyone else to see just now, and it will be nice to have a bit of a chat.'

When Susan sat down Angie said: 'I get the feeling that something is the matter; you seem different somehow.'

'Yes, I suppose I am,' said Susan. 'I get so depressed, I mean, I'm only 52 and in a way I feel my life is over.'

'What do you mean "my life is over"?' asked Angie.

'Well, you know – oh, I don't know, I'm just really depressed.'

At this point Angie, who was an experienced nurse, wondered whether Susan's depression was due to more than just the arthritis. Susan's feeling that her life was over in particular made her wonder whether there was anything the matter with Susan's relationship. It certainly seemed that Susan needed to talk to someone, so she said: 'Sometimes things seem really unfair, don't they? It must be hard to come to terms with things. I wonder how you manage generally. What about your husband?'

At this Susan broke down and started to cry. After a while she told Angie that she felt so useless and guilty and how much she missed not being able to have a normal sexual relationship with George anymore. 'It's not that he is complaining, mind', she said, 'it's just that it is not right, is it, you can't expect a man of his age to give up on sex? I'm just useless.'

Now the ice had been broken, Angie encouraged Susan to talk more freely about the nature of the problem. She discovered that Susan's knees and hips were so painful that she found it very uncomfortable to lie on her back during intercourse, and that actual penetration was very painful. Angie was able to reasssure Susan that these problems were not unsuperable and gave her some practical advice. She gave Susan a leaflet which explained a variety of different positions which would reduce the stress on the knees and hip, and told her that many people experiment with positions until they find some that suit. She also wondered whether Susan had developed Sjögren's syndrome, which is a condition that affects more than a quarter of all people with arthritis. The main symptoms of Sjögren's syndrome are dry eyes, mouth and vagina. After checking with the GP, this appreared indeed to be the case, so she gave Susan a tube of water-based lubricant to lubricate her vagina. She also said that it might be an idea to take a pain-relieving drug one hour before intercourse and to have a warm, relaxing bath.

Two days later Angie happened to meet Susan in the street and was struck how different she looked. When she commented on this

Susan said 'Yes, I feel great. Your suggestions certainly worked.I now feel that I have a new lease of life and George is very pleased too.'

Discussion

Susan's story shows how important it is for nurses to pick up clues from patients, and how easy it can be to help, provided we have the information. However, even if we do not have the information the patient needs, having identified the problem areas is the first step, and we can then set about obtaining the information or referring the patient on to someone who can help. In any case, just being listened to helps a great deal, especially as people with arthritis and other disabilities may have a low self-esteem and feel somehow less attractive and less valuable than others.

Susan's problem of painful joints, making intercourse uncomfortable, is very common among people with arthritis. Like Susan and George, people often have no experience of positions other than the missionary position, with the man on top and the couple facing each other. However, as Susan found, that position can be a real strain on a woman's back and knees. When giving people advice on different positions it is important to bear in mind that this may seem at first very strange to them. They may think it is not quite nice, if not downright kinky, and may need reassurance on this point. People may be helped to see that, provided both partners are happy, there is no reason why one position should be more acceptable than another. The main thing is good communication; partners must be honest with each other and say what they do and do not enjoy, and what causes pain or discomfort. A positive approach should be adopted. If one position does not work, then people can try another until they find a position that suits.

Some possible positions

- First of all, there is no law that says people have to be lying down; standing, kneeling, crouching or sitting down are all possibilities, either face to face, or with the man behind the woman.
- Woman on top, either lying, kneeling across the man's hips, facing the man. Alternatively, the woman may sit upright with her back to the man.
- Woman lying on her front across the bed, with perhaps a cushion under her groin and the man standing behind her between her legs, which he may support. This position is useful for people where contact causes problems.
- A variation of this position is the woman lying on her front with the man on top, supporting himself on his elbows.

So, people may like to experiment with any combination of either one partner, or both, standing, sitting, crouching or lying down Whichever position is chosen very much depends on the individuals concerned, and on what causes the least discomfort and gives the most enjoyment.

Alternatives to trying out different positions may also be considered, such as mutual masturbation or oral sex. Stroking and fondling, with or without sexual intercourse, can also give a great deal of pleasure, as potentially the whole of the body can be an erogenous zone. People may like to give each other a massage, using a pleasantly perfumed oil and using their intuition to discover what feels good. If the hands are too deformed to use them effectively, it may be possible to use a massage roller. Certainly the partner may derive as much pleasure from giving a massage as the person receiving it. Some people may benefit from sex aids, particularly if they do not have a partner but do need to obtain some sexual relief. Aids also exist to help overcome erectile problems.

A useful organization for people to contact is SPOD, the Association to Aid the Sexual and Personal Relationships of People with a Disability. The address may be found in Appendix B, Useful Addresses, at the back of the book. SPOD provides a variety of leaflets with useful and practical information.

The information contained in this section pertains not only to arthritis but to all kinds of disabilities where problems arise due to some mechanical difficulty. Also, although the information has been given with heterosexual people in mind, with a little adaptation, most is equally relevant to gay people, whether they are male or female.

CANCER

Being diagnosed as having cancer is an extremely traumatic event. After the initial shock, people's primary concern is survival as there is often still the belief that if you have cancer you are going to die. However, people's preoccupation with survival should not be taken to mean that sexuality is unimportant.

Sheila

Sheila was a 24-year-old woman who had recently got married to Dave. She had been suffering with headaches for several weeks, and at first assumed that it was migraine. Her mother tended to suffer from migraine so she thought that perhaps she was developing it too. However, when the headaches did not abate after three weeks, but became worse and were unresponsive to pain relief, she went to visit her GP. The GP had her admitted to the local hospital where she had a number of investigations, and a brain tumour was diagnosed.

Sheila and Dave were devastated. It did not seem to make any sense; after all, their lives were only just beginning. However, the surgeon thought that she had a 50% chance of survival if he operated, provided the surgery was followed by chemotherapy. Sheila was an easy-going person with a naturally optimistic outlook on life and she put a very brave front on this, especially with regards to Dave. One night, however, she was found sobbing her heart out by Denise, an agency nurse who was just doing one night-shift and had not met Sheila before. Denise was in her 40s, and worked for the agency because, having been out of nursing for a while, that was the only work she was able to get. On finding Sheila she sat down on the bed and at first said nothing but waited for Sheila to talk. When Sheila became quieter she asked her: 'What is troubling you, Sheila, why are you so upset?' She expected Sheila to talk about the cancer and being afraid to die, as that remained a real possibility. Sheila, however, told Denise that she was so incredibly worried about what all this would do to her relationship with Dave. She was not really considering dying but, as she said, 'Will he still fancy me when I have lost my hair and look absolutely awful? Maybe he will not want me anymore. Anyway I have been told that I may feel quite ill after the operation and during treatment, so I expect making love is out of the question. I just dread to think what that is going to do to our relationship.'

Discussion

You may be taken aback that a person whose life hangs in the balance is concerned with her sexual relationship. Denise certainly was. However, it does show how important the issue is and how much sexuality is a part of everything a person is.

In fact, because of the seriousness of the disease and the often drastic nature of any treatment, people with cancer are often very concerned with effects on their sexuality. If they are in a relationship they may worry, like Sheila, that they will become unattractive or even distasteful to their partner. However, whether or not they have a partner, people may worry about what the disease and treatment will do to them. Also, people may wonder whether having sexual relations is actually going to have an adverse effect on the illness.

Clearly, there are many issues that people worry about and need help with. However, because of the taboo nature of the subject, and because nurses and doctors are traditionally seen as being concerned only with the nature of the disease and its treatment, people may not feel that they can broach the subject. It is therefore doubly important for nurses to be aware of this, and certainly to be open to any cues the patient may give.

In addition, people need to be given specific information about what the disease and treatment will do them generally; talking to them about sexual effects is therefore really only part of that. After giving the patient information about their particular treatment, it is good practice to leave space for them to ask any questions. 'We have talked quite a bit, but I wonder whether there is anything you would like to ask that we haven't touched on yet?' This kind of open-ended question, particularly if the nurse gives the impression that she has plenty of time to discuss whatever it is that comes up, may give the patient the permission they feel they need to talk about any worries related to sexuality. That is what happened when Denise asked Sheila what was troubling her in the above scenario. If people do not mention anything, a sentence such as, 'I wonder what effects you feel all this may have on your relationship with your wife', or a more general statement such as, 'People are often worried how this type of treatment may affect their sexuality. What about you? I wonder whether you would like to talk about anything', puts the subject on the agenda, as it were, and gives people the opportunity to talk.

How the disease and its treatment will affect people varies greatly, depending on which parts of the body are affected, the nature and severity of the particular cancer, and the treatment chosen. Also, people react very differently physically, psychologically and emotionally.

Body image will be affected, no matter which part of the body is involved, and the patient may well grieve for the loss of the previously healthy body, particularly in the case of surgery. If the surgery is mutilating, this grief process is profound, as the damage to the body is permanent and they will never again be restored to their previous wholeness. If the surgery affects sexual organs, such as the genital areas or breast, the effect on how people perceive themselves sexually is profound. Because they fear being rejected by their partner, or in order to forestall any possible signs of distaste, some people may pretend that the treatment for the disease has made them frigid or impotent. This indicates how important it is that people are given the opportunity to talk about sexual matters. Nurses can help by letting people express how they feel and by helping them to see that this type of avoidance strategy is likely to hurt and damage the relationship more than confronting the issue. While people are feeling unwell their libido is very likely to be reduced, yet they still need physical contact, such as hugs and cuddles, support and love.

Treatments such as chemotherapy and radiotherapy may leave people feeling very tired and weak. They often suffer from nausea and pain, all of which will diminish their body image and self-esteem, and affect the way they feel as sexual beings. In addition to grief because of loss of body image, people may also have a variety of emotional responses to having cancer. Fear and anxiety about what is going to happen is the most common emotion, but some people are also angry, guilty or experience shame.

Recent 'new age' philosophies regarding the importance of a positive outlook on life, and its relevance to prevention as well as cure of cancer, have on occasion led people to believe that they are somehow 'to blame' for having cancer. Whereas it appears to be the case that a determination to get better can sometimes have beneficial effects on the disease, possibly through enhancement of the immune system, not enough is yet known about the interplay between body and mind to state that there is a direct 'cause and effect' relationship. Certainly it is unhelpful to blame people for getting ill, or for not fighting it enough. Sometimes people may be distressed because they see getting cancer as punishment for something they have done. If this is the case they may need help from someone sharing their own spiritual outlook. Having cancer is devastating enough without such additional burdens, and people should therefore be helped to see that cancer may affect anybody, even very young children, and that to see it as a punishment is inappropriate.

When men get ill they may feel guilty as they are no longer able to fulfil their role as provider for their family. They often experience a serious illness, such as cancer, as an affront to their masculinity and as a result they feel less of a man. The reduction in body image and self-esteem is made very much worse if their ability to function sexually is also affected.

Any treatment to the abdominal area, for example, whether by surgery, radio- or chemotherapy, may affect a man's ability to have and maintain an erection. However, there are great individual variations and some men do not experience any problems at all. Problems that do occur are usually temporary and improve as the affected area recovers. Sometimes this period may take months or even up to two years. It is important for people to be made aware of this and not to give up as soon as problems are encountered. The topic should therefore be very much on the agenda and be part of the normal information given to people, as it is not fair to let them find out for themselves.

Being able to maintain an erection long enough for normal intercourse to take place is very important for a man, so any failure may greatly affect his self-esteem. Penile implants may be worth considering for people where erective problems are persistent. Homosexual men, as well as other people who like to engage in anal intercourse, may be greatly disturbed by surgery on the rectum, and may need a great deal of sensitive support.

Like men, when women get ill they may also feel guilty, as they are no longer able to fulfil their role of wife and mother. They may also feel unattractive and, as was the case with Sheila, be fearful that their partner will lose interest. These fears and problems are particularly acute if the disease affects the breasts or genital area. There may also be actual physical problems regarding intercourse.

Radiotherapy to the vagina and cervix, for example, may leave scar tissue, causing the area to be less elastic. There may also be a reduction in normal natural secretions during intercourse. It is often advisable for women to have intercourse as soon as medically allowed, perhaps aided by a water-based lubricant. This is because early sexual relations prevent the tissue from becoming too tight. For women without a partner, vaginal dilation, either with the fingers or a vaginal dilator, as well as gentle masturbation may have the same effect.

As with other conditions where the body may be painful, people may like to try out various positions until they find one that suits. Initially women may find it more comfortable to be on top during intercourse as there is less pressure on her with this position and she can control the rate of penetration. Alternatively, some women prefer a side-by-side position, while facing their partner. This position may be more acceptable to some people as it is in effect only a slight variation on the missionary position, which for many people is what they are used to. Normally, unless the clitoris has been removed, the ability to experience orgasm is not affected.

Dorothy

Dorothy is a 42-year-old community worker with a husband, Derek, and two adolescent sons. Derek was the first to discover that Dorothy had a lump in her right breast. They both realized the significance immediately and Dorothy visited her doctor the next day. She knew that breast lumps are often benign, and in fact one of her friends had already undergone three lumpectomies, each time for a benign tumour. However, although she remained optimistic she was nevertheless rather worried, particularly as she realized that she had actually not been feeling quite herself lately. Dorothy's misgivings proved correct and her tumour was found to be malignant, so she had a lumpectomy followed by a year of radiotherapy and chemotherapy.

Dorothy had always been an active woman, so it was important to her to return to a normal life as soon as possible after her discharge from hospital following the operation. As she and Derek had always had a reasonably active sex life, getting back to normal included for Dorothy the resumption of normal sexual relations with her husband. Derek was very supportive and did not pressurize her in any way, but Dorothy became very upset about her inability to experience any pleasure from making love. She felt physical as well as mental pain every time they tried and could not understand this as it was her breast, not her genital area which had been affected. In fact, as she told her doctor, she felt numb from the waist downwards and wondered whether her loss of libido was due to the medication she was still taking. Her doctor assured her that this was unlikely to be the case and that her sexual feelings would return in time. Meanwhile he referred her to Margaret, the practice counsellor. Margaret was an ex-nurse and had counselled many women following mastectomy and helped Dorothy to see that her problems were emotional rather than physical.

At first, Dorothy resisted this idea; she regarded herself as a strong woman who would not let things get her down. Also, because of her job, she was well aware of the way in which grief can affect people and had indeed often helped people herself. She did not think she had any 'hang-ups' about her scar and was not afraid to undress in front of Derek. Also, the mastectomy counsellor at the hospital had been instrumental in her finding a suitable prosthesis, so she was not too worried about her external appearance. However, Dorothy came to realize that just because she thought she was coping so well and wanted to be so strong, she had not allowed herself to grieve. Actually, she had had a very traumatic time in the last year, losing both her parents, and her sister had had breast cancer the year before. With Margaret's help, Dorothy realized that there is no shame attached to being affected by such experiences. In a way she had undergone a real battering physically as well as emotionally, and it was not surprising that this affected her libido. After all, as she said herself later, there is only so much a person can take – nobody is superhuman.

A year later Dorothy felt much better in herself although, due to the medication, she had put on a great deal of weight which naturally made her feel less sexually attractive. Another effect of the medication was that it stopped her menstruation, which she experienced as another loss in her view of herself as a woman. However, she found that she was now able to enjoy sexual relations with Derek approximately once every three weeks. Although before the operation they had had intercourse on a more frequent basis, she felt optimistic that in time she would be back to normal. In a way Dorothy realizes that she is one of the lucky ones. 'If Derek had not been so supportive I doubt whether our marriage would have lasted,' she said.

Discussion

Dorothy's story illustrates just how traumatic a mastectomy can be for a woman, even if she is supposed to be cured, and how the effects are not always predictable. It is important for nurses to be aware of this as breast cancer is very common, and in 1990 caused 13 000 deaths in the United Kingdom alone. This makes it the second highest cause of death for people under the age of 65, after heart disease (HMSO, 1991).

Activity 7

Like Dorothy, it is estimated that approximately one-third of women experience sexual problems following mastectomy, and that a quarter suffer from anxiety or depression (Maguire *et al.*, 1978).

What do you think are possible reasons for this high proportion of women who experience emotional and/or sexual problems?

Discussion

In a way, the breast is very much a symbol of a woman's femininity and is bound up intimately with her identity and self-concept. A woman who has lost all or part of her breast, or whose breast has been altered in some way, may therefore feel diminished in her femininity. In our culture, as well as in many others, breasts are a symbol of female sexuality as well as of motherhood. 'Men-only' magazines and certain popular newspapers feature attractive young women with perfectly shaped, usually fairly large, breasts. Because of this emphasis on breasts it is often the case that flat-chested women somehow feel inferior and less desirable sexually, hence the practice of breast enlarging operations. If flat-chested women can feel inferior, it is not surprising that women whose breast has been mutilated in some way feel very much worse. Also, because of the high incidence of mortality, many women obviously also fear a recurrence of the cancer.

Initially, women often fear rejection by their partner and will not let them look at the breast. Some women may themselves initially be very afraid to look at the scar. This is where nurses can help. If a woman is experiencing these problems, they can be helped to understand that their reaction is normal and shared by many other women. It may also help them to know that people's imagination is often very much worse than the reality, and people are often helped by looking at the scar in a supportive environment.

In Dorothy's case the mastectomy counsellor was present when Dorothy and Derek together looked at her breast for the first time, which greatly helped Dorothy to the extent that she did not mind undressing in front of Derek. Dorothy was fortunate in that her breasts had not diminished in sensitivity, which is what can happen to some women. If they liked to include stimulation of the breast as part of love-making, then such diminished sensitivity can be distressing. Sometimes a sexual counsellor can help people feel better about themselves and explore alternative ways of giving each other sexual pleasure.

Rhea

How nurses behave towards women who have had a mastectomy may be crucial. Rhea had been worried about her breast lump for a while, but had not mentioned it to anyone in the hope that it would go away. Her relationship with her boyfriend Peter was rocky anyway and she felt she really did not need any more problems. However, she began to lose weight to the extent that other people were commenting on it. Rhea realized that she could bury her head in the sand no longer and went to her doctor. Unfortunately, her reluctance to seek medical help meant that a rather large part of her breast needed to be removed. This totally devastated her. She felt sure Peter would find her repulsive and so she refused to see him. Her hospital did not have a mastectomy counsellor and the nurses on the ward were, on the whole, young and inexperienced. Because Rhea put a brave face on things while she was in hospital, no-one really realized how upset she was, and apart from being given a leaflet and a temporary prosthesis, she received no support at all.

On discharge, Rhea became very unhappy and depressed; she missed Peter terribly but was convinced that she had made the right decision. She could not see how he could possibly still want her after her, as she saw it, mutilation. Peter, for his part, was upset too. He had no idea of what she was going through and assumed that she no longer loved him. Rhea found that she needed constant reassurance. Rather than hiding the scar, as many women would, she felt a compulsive need to show it to people, whether they wanted to see it or not. She did this because she needed constant reassurance that she was still attractive and that the scar was not as bad as she felt it was. When she showed her scar Rhea scoured people's faces for any sign of revulsion and was thrown in deep depression if she thought that people did show any distaste.

Finally, her best friend realized that things were not going well, and urged Rhea to seek professional help. Rhea refused, saying that she did not need help, and anyway what could anyone do? Then, by chance, she met Patricia, who had also had a mastectomy and appeared to be coping very well. Feeling that finally here was someone who could understand, Rhea broke down, cried for a long time and poured her heart out to Patricia. Patricia just let her talk as she realized that was what Rhea needed, and afterwards said that she had gone through many of the same emotions. Although her relationship with her boyfriend was good now, her anxiety, depression and loss of interest sexually had initially created problems. Now, however, as she told Rhea, their relationship was stronger than ever and they were planning to get married. 'Go and see Peter', she urged Rhea. 'You have nothing to lose. It seems to me that you cannot be unhappier than you are now. Why deprive yourself of a chance of happiness?' Rhea took some persuading – she was actually terrified of Peter's reaction – but eventually went to see him. As soon as they saw each other, they fell into each other's arms and realized that they still loved each other and would work things out.

Discussion

Rhea was lucky to have found an understanding woman with the same experience and a boyfriend who was able to love and support her after all. However, her problems could have been very much minimized if she had received more help, support and information while in hospital. In addition to having an opportunity to talk about her feelings and express any anxieties, she could have been given the names and addresses of a few counsellors and self-help organizations. Not all women need to see a professional to help them come to terms with what has happened to them. Many, like Rhea, will resist this idea but are happy to talk to people who have had the same experience. (A number of self-help organizations are included in Appendix B, at the back of the book.)

PROSTATECTOMY

Ivor

Ivor is a 52-year-old man who works for a publishing company. He was divorced 15 years ago and has three grown-up children, none of whom live with him. Since his divorce he has had a number of longish relationships, each lasting four years or so, but now he is not interested in anything permanent. 'I have been disappointed too often,' he says. 'Mind you, I love women, I just do not want to live with them. Anyway, variety keeps you interested.' Ivor is very gregarious and women do find him attractive. Despite the lack of any serious girlfriends, therefore, he does have quite an active sex life.

Ivor realized that something was wrong when he began getting up at night to pass urine. This was new as he usually slept right through until the alarm woke him. At first it was just once or twice a night, but lately he seemed to get up all the time. Ivor felt this was interfering with his sex life as his girlfriends were wondering what was going on. After a particularly sleepless night, which had particularly annoyed the woman he was with, he decided to do something about it and went to see his GP. The GP referred him to the local urologist and afer a number of investigations an enlarged prostate was diagnosed, necessitating an operation.

Ivor was rather worried about this and wondered whether it would have an effect on his ability to function sexually. Because he appeared very jovial and confident the nurses on the unit did not think he was worried and just gave him the standard advice regarding coming into hospital. Because of his connections in the publishing world Ivor was able to seek out quite a bit of relevant reading material, and by the time his operation was due he probably knew more than some of the staff. He had learned that, although in the vast majority of cases libido and the ability to perform sexually is not affected, there were a few unlucky men who were adversely affected. He realized that it depended on the type of operation and therefore insisted the surgeon explained exactly to him which operation would be used.

The operation was a success and on recovery he was rather anxious to try out whether he was still as he put it 'a man'. He did not say anything to Ceri, a woman whom he knew only casually and who knew nothing about his hospital stint, and was rather relieved to find that everything was still in working order. 'I do not know what I would have done if it had not been all right,' he said later. 'I really don't know that I could have coped with that.'

Discussion

Although Ivor's story had a happy ending, it does indicate how nurses can never know whether people are worried or not and must see it as part of their role to place sexual consequences of surgery on the agenda. In other words, it is part of the nurse's role to broach the subject; it cannot be assumed that a patient is not worried, does not want to know or knows the facts already. Ivor was fortunate in that he had the ways and means of getting the information he needed. However, many patients would not be in that position and might end up worrying needlessly.

As Ivor found out, libido and the ability to achieve orgasm are not usually affected following a prostatectomy, especially if the transurethral route is used. Patients should be warned, though, that their urine may have a milky appearance at times due to retrograde ejaculation of the seminal fluid into the bladder. Another consequence of this is infertility. However, benign enlargement of the prostate is a condition normally associated with the older male, for whom infertility is not normally a problem.

In cases of malignancy, a radical prostatectomy may be performed, which includes removal of the seminal vesicles so that there will be no ejaculation of semen. The capacity to achieve an orgasm is not normally affected, although some men do experience erectile problems which may on occasion be permanent. Artificial erection aids or penile implants may be advised for people in this category.

DIABETES

Kevin

Kevin is an 18-year-old trainee welder with a fine physique. He is a star in his local rugby team and likes to keep himself in good shape. However, he is very gregarious, likes pubbing, clubbing and going to discos. He has no steady girlfriend, but he is popular with the opposite sex and at the moment he tends to change his girlfriends frequently. Kevin was diagnosed as having diabetes recently, necessitating twice daily injections of insulin.

While in hospital to stabilize his diabetes, Kevin was having a practice session with his primary nurse, Fiona, on giving himself injections. Kevin appeared reluctant and uninterested, so Fiona thought she would leave it for that day, assuming that he was just feeling a bit 'off'. The next day she tried again, but there was no change, Kevin did not seem to pick up what she was telling him and gave every impression of not wanting to know. 'What is the matter, Kevin?' asked Fiona. 'You are a bright lad, yet you do not seem to want to learn about your injections. Surely you are not squeamish.' 'No, definitely not,' snapped Kevin, 'but now I'm no better than a bloody junky, am I, needing injections all the time?'

Fiona was taken aback. 'No you're not,' she said. 'That's entirely different. What makes you say that?' Then Kevin told her that he was the second eldest of the family, but that his older brother was a drug addict, always in trouble for obtaining money from people and generally making a complete mess of his life. 'I always vowed that I would never have anything to do with drugs whatsoever,' Kevin said, 'But look at me now, I am no better than he is. I cannot live without my fix. What girls are going to be interested in a bloke like me who needs injections to stay alive? I'm just not worth the bother; this is no way for a bloke to live. I work out, I train, I play rugby, I've always been strong and healthy. In fact, I have done everything

I possibly could to avoid becoming like him. I also want my parents to be proud of me. What is there to be proud of now? It's not fair, why did this have to happen to me?'

After this explosion of feelings, which had been bottled up for a while, it took a great deal of talking, listening and counselling before Kevin began to start to come to terms with the idea of having diabetes. At his age it was a devastating thing to happen, totally changing how he saw himself and greatly affecting his body image and self-esteem. Also, having to come to terms with a life-long condition instead of being a normal, healthy man is very difficult for anyone to cope with, particularly at such a young age. In Kevin's case the grief reaction was very much intensified by the fact that he thought he had ended up just like his brother, which was something he had tried to avoid at all costs.

Discussion

Kevin was not unusual in having a severe emotional reaction to having been diagnosed as a diabetic; many people find it very difficult to come to terms with. However, it is very important that people do come to accept their condition as they are more likely to comply with the changes in lifestyle that it requires. There are a great many problems that people can develop such as eye conditions, hypertension and infections in the limbs which, if neglected, sometimes necessitate amputation. The better people adhere to their diet and drug treatment, the less likely their blood sugar levels are to fluctuate and the less the damage to their body will be. As far as sexuality is concerned, the only effect for women seems to be that they tend to be more prone to vaginal infections. For men, in cases of severe diabetes, there is the possibility of impotence and infertility, probably caused by vascular and neurological damage. However, by adhering to the prescribed treatment and seeking medical advice as soon as the diabetes appears to become unstable, the likelihood of developing problems of infertility and impotence can be reduced.

MULTIPLE SCLEROSIS

Barry

Barry is a 45-year-old single, homosexual man who developed multiple sclerosis two years ago. Initially he resolved to fight the disease and tried out many diets and other remedies, but all to no avail. This gave him a feeling of uselessness and of being out of control. It greatly affected how he saw himself as a man; he felt a 'waste of time' and certainly not worthy of anyone's attention.

While having a few days in hospital he became quite friendly with Ivor, the charge nurse. Ivor had done a counselling course and was particularly interested in the existentialist approach (van Deurzen-Smith, 1988). He helped Barry realize that although he could not really influence the course of the illness, he did have a choice about how to react to it. 'This is where our personal freedom really lies,' he told Barry. 'No matter what the situation, we are always free to choose our attitude towards it; we always have a choice. You can choose to be pessimistic and depressed; that's your choice. Maybe you even need to do that from time to time, after all, it is a real blow to develop MS and you do need to grieve. But you can also choose to be, on the whole, optimistic – to take each day as it comes, and to enjoy all the pleasures, no matter how small, that come your way.' Barry was quiet for a long time. 'Thanks, Ivor, it sounds good. I need to think about this; I'm not sure I can quite take all this on board at the moment.'

Somehow, as Barry said later, that conversation with Ivor was a turning point in his life. Gradually he became less angry and more accepting of himself and his situation. He became much easier to get on with, which greatly benefited his relationship with Trevor, his partner of two years. Trevor went to see Ivor and told him that Barry and he were now getting on well. He realized that he had initially been overprotective of Barry, and had been too quick to come to his aid with the result that Barry felt reduced as a man.

'It's not easy, Ivor, to see him struggle, but he wants to do whatever he can, even if it takes a long time and tires him. I respect him for that and I know that when it does get too much for him he will tell me. In a way our relationship is much better than that of many other gays. I used to be quite selfish but now let Barry take the lead and decide when he wants to have sex as he needs to take it easy for a while beforehand to reserve his energies. Also, we have discovered how nice it is to just caress and hug each other. In a way you could say that as far as our relationship is concerned, we are actually quite lucky.'

Discussion

Barry and Trevor's situation is not really very different from that of heterosexual couples where one partner has MS. Like Barry, some women may also be fiercely independent and resent being wrapped in cottonwool. It is very important not to forget the well partner and give them an opportunity to talk about their situation and express any grief, sadness and worries they may feel. Sadly, if a relationship is already rocky, one of the partners developing a disease like MS does not always bring the couple closer together. For some it may be too much of a strain and the well partner may leave or, while staying in the relationship, develop interests in other people.

DRUGS

How often do we, as nurses, tell patients all about the drugs they are taking, as well as the most common side-effects to watch out for? Probably not enough. Yet most drugs have side-effects that the patient should know about. Failure to inform them may cause much distress, especially as the patient may not realize that whatever symptoms they are experiencing are due to the drug. Many drugs have an effect on sexuality, and it should really be part of normal nursing care to inform patients of this. There is also the issue of informed consent. Would a patient agree to take a drug that makes it likely that he will lose much of his interest in sex? The answer may be yes or no, depending on how serious is the condition that the drug is prescribed for. However, the patient should have the choice.

It is impossible to list here individually all the drugs which affect sexuality, and in any case such a list would soon be out of date as new drugs come onto the market continuously. So, in order to know the possible effects of a drug on sexuality as well as other side-effects, nurses should make it part of their normal routine to check in the *British National Formulary* for that type of information.

However, it is possible to some extent to group drugs together with regard to sexuality-affecting side-effects. The list below sets out some of the most common effects and the drugs which cause them.

Decreased libido

- diuretics
- antihypertensives
- antihistamines
- corticosteroids
- tranquillizers/sedatives

Women

Amenorrhoea

- cytotoxics
- diuretics

Decreased vaginal lubrication

- antihistamines

Men

Decreased sperm count

- corticosteroids
- cytotoxics

Impotence

- diuretics
- tranquillizers/sedatives
- antidepressants
- antihistamines
- antihypertensives
- corticosteroids

CONCLUSION

The conditions discussed in this chapter are not the only ones to affect people's sexuality, nor do the examples given discuss the only way in which people react. As mentioned at the beginning of this chapter, sexuality is very much a part of who we are, and any illness, or condition or disability therefore will affect it. The important issue is for the topic to be on the agenda at all times, and for nurses to realize that sexuality is an important part of people and therefore definitely falls within the remit of holistic nursing care.

The examples discussed all indicate the importance of good listening skills. However, this is exactly what nurses sometimes find very difficult. Pure training is very much geared to the practical and nurses often feel that they 'must do something'. Although sometimes there is definitely something nurses can do, they must beware of jumping in with advice too soon. Sometimes patients really need time to express how they feel and what troubles them.

'All nurses can counsel' is a phrase often heard. 'We all do it all the time, it comes with experience, doesn't it?' It is true that some people seem to be more naturally inclined to be good listeners and to be able to say the right thing. More often than not, however, nurses jump in with giving advice, which may at that moment not be what the person needs. They may be well aware of all the things they could try and do not need someone else to tell them. What they do need at such a time, though, is to be heard. They need someone to care enough to take the time to listen to their story. This is not to say that nurses should not give advice. Of course we should, it is very much part of our role. There is, however, a time and place for everything;

jumping in too soon with reassurance and advice may be perceived by the patient as rejection, and evidence of not being taken seriously.

Nurses who decide to undertake counselling training often say that not immediately coming up with a solution is one of the hardest things they have to learn. Although many nurses now have some idea of counselling skills, there is a real difference between using counselling skills and counselling. Sometimes, a nurse who has learned the skills of paraphrasing, reflection and asking open questions may find herself in a situation where the patient has been encouraged to 'open up' and talk about their feelings. However, having done so, the nurse may then be at a loss as to what to do next. 'I wish I'd never learned these skills', said Pat, a student nurse. 'I was at a complete loss and felt quite panicky when a patient told me a lot of things. Help, now what do I do, I thought.' Pat realized that she was out of her depth and with the patient's permission talked to Andrea, a staff nurse who was undertaking a Diploma in Counselling. As Andrea explained to Pat, she helped the patient to explore and clarify issues that worried her, and helped her to find her own solutions. In fact, her reason for undertaking counselling training was that she had had experiences similar to Pat, but at the time there had been no-one to turn to, which left her with a feeling of somehow having failed the patient. It is unlikely that the patient thought so, though; just being listened to is often all they want and expect. It is probably nurses' own feelings of 'having to do something' that makes them feel inadequate.

It is important for nurses to realize their own limitations, and not to take on more than they can cope with, and to know when to refer on and to whom. A knowledge of useful people and organizations in one's own area and relevant to the specialty wherein one works is therefore essential. Leaflets with this kind of information should be available on all wards and in doctors' surgeries. Many nurses now realize this and are developing leaflets and booklets on a variety of topics and conditions, often as part of post-registration courses and projects. This, as well as the interest shown by many nurses in developing their counselling role, is very encouraging and indicative of the integrity and enthusiasm with which many nurses approach their role.

REFERENCES

The Guardian (1990) You're never too old, 7 February.
HMSO (1991) *On the State of the Public Health for the Year 1990*, HMSO, London.

Maguire, P. *et al.* (1978) Psychiatric problems in the first year after mastectomy. *British Medical Journal,* **279**, 963–5.

Masters, W.H. and Johnson, V.E. (1966) *Human Sexual Response,* Little, Brown & Co., Boston.

Rogers, C. (1980) *A Way of Being,* Houghton Mifflin, Boston, Massachusetts.

Roper, N., Logan, W.W. and Tierney, A.J. (1980) *The Elements of Nursing,* Churchill Livingstone, Edinburgh.

Stockwell, F. (1972) *The Unpopular Patient,* Royal College of Nursing, London.

Van Deurzen-Smith, E. (1988) *Existential Counselling in Practice,* Sage Publications, London.

FURTHER READING

Bancroft, J. (1989) *Human Sexuality and its Problems,* 2nd edn, Churchill Livingstone, Edinburgh.

Brown, H. and Craft, A. (1989) *Thinking the Unthinkable,* FPA Education Unit.

Bullard, D.G. and Knight, S.E. (eds) (1981) *Sexuality and Physical Disability; Personal Perspectives,* Mosby, St Louis.

Cancerlink (1988) *Body Image, Sexuality and Cancer,* Cancerlink, London.

Cole, B. and Dryden, W. (eds) (1988) *Sex Therapy in Britain,* Open University Press, Milton Keynes.

Connell, H. (1983) More than a physical illness. Multiple sclerosis management. *Nursing Mirror,* 79(24), 15 June, 40–1.

Davis, H. and Fallowfield, L. (eds) (1991) *Counselling and Communication in Health Care,* John Wiley, Chichester.

Gibson, H.B. (1992) *The Emotional and Sexual Lives of Older People,* Chapman & Hall, London.

Greengross, W. (1976) *Entitled to Love: The Sexual and Emotional Needs of the Handicapped,* Mallaby Press and National Marriage Guidance Council, in association with the National Fund for Research into Crippling Diseases.

Greengross, W. and Greengross, S. (1989) *Living, Loving and Aging,* Age Concern, London.

Hawton, K. (1985) *Sex Therapy, A Practical Guide,* Jason Aronson Inc., Northvale, New Jersey.

Money, T. (1975) *Sexual Options for Paraplegics and Quadraplegics,* Little, Brown & Co., Boston.

Skrine, R.L. (ed) (1989) *Introduction to Psychosexual Medicine,* Montana Press, Carlisle.

Spense, S.H. (1991) *Psychosexual Therapy. A Cognitive–Behavioural Approach,* Chapman & Hall, London.

Stewart, W. (1985) *Counselling in Rehabilitation,* Croom Helm, Beckenham.

Tunnadine, L.P.D. (1983) *The Making of Love,* Cape, London.

Webb, A. (1989) *Experiences of Hysterectomy,* Optima, in association with the Hysterectomy Support Group, London.

Webb, C. (1985) *Sexuality, Nursing and Health,* John Wiley, Chichester.

CHAPTER 8

Case studies

I could not trust you with my thoughts and apprehensions, there was so much I needed to say, but couldn't. I could not show the love I felt for Paul because I feared your remarks. So many times I wanted Paul to hold me, to cry with me, lie with me, but my hesitation was your creation. All my life I had to battle to be me. AIDS wore me down and I had no strength left to fight you.

Case 7, page 172

LEARNING OBJECTIVES

After reading this chapter you should be able to:

1. appreciate how the concept of sexuality can be affected during illness, or by conditions;
2. identify differing attitudes and values to sexuality;
3. discuss possible helping actions and behaviours when sexuality has been compromised.

FOR DISCUSSION AND ROLE-PLAY

The following case studies are fictitious accounts; if they bear any relationship to actual events it is purely coincidental. The studies are presented as a basis for discussion or as possible role-play situations. The cases could be utilized within a programme of study or a workshop setting. Their use could help to cement understanding and demonstrate application to practice. Actual or potential problems are highlighted, together with suggested helping strategies. It would be foolhardy to propose that the identified problem/s and concurrent helping strategies are exhaustive and conclusive. Each case is unique. What is offered here is a point of view, to which various alternatives could be suggested.

Case 1: All tied up

Dave is 22 years old, single, and employed as a carpenter and joiner for a local builder. He enjoys life to the full. He has had a steady girlfriend for the past three years. He still lives with his parents, but spends most of his free time out with his girlfriend. Thursday night, however, is reserved for a night out with the lads. He has one passionate hobby – motorbikes.

On his way to work Dave was involved in a road traffic accident, he lost control of his motorbike and crashed into an oncoming vehicle. As a result of the accident he fractured both femurs, a humerus, four ribs and his pelvis. Since the accident he has been nursed on the same orthopaedic ward. He has been confined to bed for the past six weeks on traction. He is making steady progress, and all his fractures are healing well.

The staff have found him to be an outgoing person, always ready with a joke. However, the staff are becoming increasingly annoyed by his suggestive remarks, and occasional over-zealous touching. Staff are now starting to avoid him, and there have been a number of complaints to the nurse in charge.

Try to answer the following questions.

1. Is this normal behaviour?
2. Why is Dave behaving in this way?
3. What has caused this behaviour?
4. How should the situation be handled? Imagine you were going to talk to Dave about his behaviour, what would you say? (Try role-playing the scene.)

Case 2: Turn off the light, dear

Ann Thorpe, aged 42, has been happily married for 20 years, and has two children. Two weeks ago she visited her GP complaining of pain in her left breast. The results identified carcinoma, and she was admitted for a mastectomy. The operation and subsequent postoperative period was uneventful.

A week after leaving hospital, Ann was back at her doctor's in a very distressed state. The doctor found that Ann was too afraid to show her husband the scar, and too scared to resume any sexual activity. In fact, for the past week Ann had been getting changed in the bathroom before going to bed, just so that her husband did not see the scar. Before the operation, they had both enjoyed sexual intimacy and intercourse.

Try answering the following questions.

1. What action could have been taken in hospital to help avoid this situation?
2. Why is Ann feeling the way she is?
3. What can be done to help?

Case 3: I want a girlfriend

Jim is 20 years old and has Down's syndrome. He has no close family, and has lived in institutionalized care since he was five. He is making steady progress in social and domestic skills. He has a job in the sheltered workshop, where he makes packing cases for a removal company. He has a mental age of a 12-year-old.

For the past three years staff have been working towards Jim moving out into the community. He has spent a number of weekends in sheltered accommodation with no major problems. It all looks set for Jim to move out into a hostel, yet one aspect is causing reservations about the move. Jim has been insistent about getting a girlfriend when he moves out, and 'living the life of a bachelor', as he puts it.

Try answering the following questions.

1. Should there be any restrictions on Jim's proposed sexuality?
2. If Jim is to go out into the community, what and how should he be told about sexuality?

Case 4: Dirty old man

Percy Walker is a 70-year-old, retired headmaster. He has a right hemiplegia, and is being nursed on a rehabilitation ward, which has physiotherapy and occupational suites attached. Since his admission three weeks ago he has made good progress, regaining some movement in his right arm, and is now able to stand using a Zimmer frame. He is a likable man with excellent manners. However, there have been instances (which are increasing in number) when he touches people inappropriately, and makes explicit sexual undertones.

Try answering the following questions.

1. Is this behaviour acceptable?
2. What should be done about Percy's behaviour?

Case 5: Stiff hips

Mary Lewis has suffered with rheumatoid arthritis for the past 10 years. She is at the peak of available treatments. She is married with a devoted husband, and has three daughters. At the age of 45 she still considers herself to be sexually active and attractive. However, over the past year her ability to enjoy sex has been hampered by pain in her hips. This affects her ability to have and enjoy sexual intercourse. Repercussions of this diminished aspect of love are making her fearful of even hugging and kissing, just in case it leads on to intercourse. Slowly this is starting to alter the marital relationship, and frustrations are starting to emerge.

Try answering the following questions.

1. Can the reduced sexual activity be attributed to the pain from the arthritis?
2. How can Mary and her husband be helped?

Case 6: The real man

Alan Bates, a 17-year-old, was admitted to the young persons ward in the early hours of the morning. He was in a semi-conscious state. Active emergency treatment was commenced, and a diagnosis of diabetes was made. The next morning Alan had made an excellent recovery, although he was still a little weary. Teaching about diabetes was quickly instigated so that Alan could start to resume some control over his condition and treatments. However, Alan seemed unenthusiastic about the whole thing, and continually needing prompting about meal and injection times. He had a lazy attitude to the whole diagnosis and care. Because of this, early discharge was planned to enable Alan to get back to his normal way of life: basically, he was left to get on with it to see how he would cope.

Three days later Alan was re-admitted because of alternating hyperglycaemia and hypoglycaemia. He was stabilized, but was still unconcerned about his condition. One day while having a conversation with the diabetic specialist Alan had a fit of anger. 'I'm fed-up of injecting myself, taking this and that to eat. What a waste of time. My mum wraps me up in cotton wool and says

I've got to do this and that. I can't go out with my mates, can't drink what I want, have to be in the house at a certain time – just in case something happens.'

Try answering the following questions:

1. Why is Alan behaving in this way?
2. Could he have been treated differently?

Case 7: A note

Mike was a 30-year-old advertisement executive with his own company. Over the last three weeks he had been losing weight, and had developed a persistent cough. He visited his GP who took an extensive history. On suspecting pneumonia, the doctor arranged for Mike to be admitted to hospital straight away.

Many tests and procedures followed. Eventually one day the doctors confirmed Mike's worst fears – he had AIDS. Mike never really recovered from the news, and visibly started to waste away.

Mike had no real family to speak of; they had cut him off' when they found out he was gay. Paul, Mike's lover for the past 12 years, was a devoted partner and visited every day. Two weeks after admission Mike died.

When nurses went to sort out his belongings they found a small note pad; in it they found the following note:

Nurses,

I have no idea why I was born gay. For the first part of my short life I suffered considerable torment from friends and family for the way I was. Yet out of the torment I learned to respect myself, and I returned the respect to others who accepted me for what I was. Some of you did not; I saw your sideways glances, the nods, and I heard the giggling in the office when Paul visited.

Was there any need for those masks, aprons and gloves every time you touched me? You avoided me when I wanted to talk; I was alone for hours. Why couldn't we have talked? Why did you assume that air of matter of fact-ness when you gave me my tablets or washed me? I could feel your cold hands.

I could not trust you with my thoughts and apprehen-sions, there was so much I needed to say, but couldn't. I could not show the love I felt for Paul because I feared your remarks. So many times I wanted Paul to hold me, to cry with me, lie with me, but my hesitation was your creation. All my life I had to battle to be me. AIDS wore me down and I had no strength left to fight you.

It's too late for me now the damage is done, but next time please remember – see me for who I am, not what I am or appear to be.

Try answering the following questions.

1. Why did some of the nurses behave the way they did?
2. Is this a true representation of how gay people are cared for?

Case 8: Everything in moderation

Ken Taylor was 43, and married with two teenage children. He had made excellent recovery from his first heart attack, and was due to go home in the next two days. Medication consisted of frusemide, antihypertensives and glycerin trinitrate.

Ken had an outgoing personality. On one occasion when he was being given his medication, he asked if he could have a quiet word. The gist of the conversation was as follows:

Ken	'These tablets I'm taking – they're all right, I mean no side-effects or anything?'
Nurse	'No, not really. The white ones are for your water works, the pink ones are for your blood pressure, and the tiny white one is to put under your tongue when you have chest pains . . . I thought the doctors had gone through this with you.'
Ken	'Oh, yes they have, but I thought I'd ask just in case.'
Nurse	'Was there something else?'
Ken	'When I go home will I be able to carry on as before?'
Nurse	'Well, yes, within reason. Just remember, everything in moderation. I'll just finish giving these tablets out and I'll get back to you.'

With this, the conversation ended and the nurse carried on with the drug round.

Try answering the following questions.

1. Do you think the nurse answered the questions adequately?

2. Was there a deeper issue which was either unidentified or avoided by the nurse?
3. Try role-playing the scene and see what happens.

Case 9: Sexually active

Jean had suffered from multiple sclerosis for the past five years. Her condition is steadily deteriorating. Every two months she is admitted to the local hospital for two weeks' respite care. This gives Len, her husband, an opportunity to rest, and catch up on his own activities. Len and Jean have been married for 20 years; they have one child, Deborah, who is 10 years old.

It was during one of the respite periods that Jean started to talk about some of the problems she was experiencing. It seemed that Jean's major concern was keeping the relationship with her husband sexually active. Before her multiple sclerosis, they had enjoyed an active and enjoyable sex life. She realized that as her condition progressed this may become more and more difficult.

Try answering the following question.

1. How should the situation be handled?

Case 10: Stressed out

John is 34 years old and married, with two children aged 10 and 12 years. His wife works as a teacher. He works as a salesman for an insurance company. His job is demanding and very stressful as the majority of his salary is dependent on sales. He works long hours well into most weekday evenings and at weekends finds it difficult to wind down. Over the last six months there have been increasing rumours that the company is going to cut back on its sales force due to financial problems and he has been working harder.

He has been to his GP and requested help with an increasing inability to sleep and feelings of panic when he is faced with meeting new clients. He has seen the GP because his wife told him to go for help. The GP suggested that John sees the male community psychiatric nurse who works at the practice and he has agreed to this. The GP has not prescribed any medication.

During the second session at the CPN's practice clinic, John says that he and his wife have been having problems in their relationship. He states that he has neither felt like nor had sexual relations with her for about three months. Prior to this they had enjoyed sexual intercourse about once or twice a week. He is worried about this situation, is embarrassed when talking about it and does not know what to do.

Try to answer the following questions.

1. What may be the reasons for John's embarrassment?
2. What may be an appropriate response to John's disclosure of the problems?
3. How may John's situation have caused or contributed to his sexual problem?
4. What would the CPN need to clarify with John during this session?
5. What issues may the CPN need to consider before the next session?

HOW DO YOUR ANSWERS COMPARE?

Case 1

1. Is his behaviour normal?

The short answer to this is yes, for him. Before his accident Dave was an active man. He had a steady girlfriend, and socialized with a group of men his own age. He is perhaps finding his condition annoying, not being able to control his very natural desires.

2. Why is Dave behaving in this way?

It is not unusual for men who have been nursed back to health to feel some sort of love and gratitude, especially if those doing the caring (which may be of an intimate nature) are young and female. It is easy to see how these emotions can be tied up with sexuality, and as such be part of sexual arousal. He may be missing his girlfriend. We have no idea of how active his sex life was before the accident.

3. What has caused this behaviour?

This is related to point 2. The result of the behaviour could be the result of Dave's socialization process – how he sees women, and what part women play in his life. The behaviour may be a result of his feelings of loss of control, that is, being bed-fast for a long period and having to rely on others (women) for support and care. His behaviour could be an effort to reinstate his role as a man.

4. How should the situation be handled? Imagine you were going to talk to Dave about his behaviour, what would you say?

There are a number of ways to handle this situation. The main occurring theme should be the expression of how the behaviour is affecting the nurse–patient relationship. An expression of roles and responsibilities should also be highlighted. There could be recognition that the behaviour is not uncommon and that the cause could be discussed. Whatever the outcome, it is important that Dave knows his behaviour is not appreciated. A telling off – 'Now this monkey business, Dave, has just got to stop' – does not help the patient in any way, and may damage the nurse–patient relationship still further. It may be an idea to allow his girlfriend some time alone with Dave, so that they can share a degree of intimacy.

Case 2

1. What action could have been taken in hospital to help avoid this situation?

Ann should have been given time and help to reflect on how the surgery was going to affect her sexuality. How did she feel about the change in body image? What effect was this now going to have on her sexual relations wiht her husband? These are obviously sensitive areas. It would appear that nurses do not initiate or enter into discussion about sexuality (Waterhouse and Metcalfe, 1991) and are not equipped to cope even if they did (Hogan, 1980). The nature and content of any discussions with Ann would have to be sensitive. A degree of empathy, support and compassion, together with some counselling and listening skills are prerequisites for taking on such discussion (see Chapter 6).There are, however, a growing number of nurse specialists (for example, breast care nurses) who may assist patients in coming to terms with change caused by surgery.

2. Why is Ann feeling the way she is?

It is impossible to multilate the body to this extent and not expect or consider possible psychological repercussions. Ann is reacting in a normal way; she is anxious and apprehensive about how her husband will react. Her feelings may fluctuate from anger to outright depression. She has changed; the association of the female breast with femininity and sexual attraction is inescapable. Ann may be experiencing threats to her womanhood and her ability to remain attractive to her husband. One must also recognize that the cancer and its possible spread may also be an undercurrent to Ann's feelings.

3. *What can be done to help?*

The nurse–patient relationship is an important factor in helping strategies. Rehabilitation starts at admission. Therefore discussions, advice and feelings are identified from the start where care and helping strategies can be instigated. The operation is going to have repercussions on both partners, therefore any discussions must involve Ann's husband. Knowledge about the operations and impending recovery are discussed; what the scar will look like, what prostheses are available, and what these look like. Feelings and anxieties are identified and talked through, with the nurse filling in uncertainties, and giving credence to the feelings.

Case 3

1. *Should there be any restrictions on Jim's proposed sexuality?*

The answer to this is not easy. There has been an increase in the desire to see those in institutions come out into the community. If we believe in the idea of normalization, then it should include the concept of sexuality. If we restrict Jim's activities or needs in any way, then it sends a contradictory message. Part of the answer to this question will reflect personal as well as society's values on sexuality and the handicapped.

2. *If Jim is to go out into the community, what and how should he be told about sexuality?*

Part of Jim's preparation for discharge should have included discussion and advice about his sexuality, and ways in which it can be expressed. To be suddenly faced with the problem of relationships and 'wanting a girlfriend' just before discharge is short-sighted. Discussion about sexuality and relationships should have taken place over a planned period of time. The whole area of sexuality and the handicapped needs careful and skilful handling. Issues of personal relationships, expression of love, appropriate sexual behaviour, sexual performance, marriage, contraception and birth control all need to be discussed. This represents a catalogue of issues that cannot be tackled in an afternoon before discharge. So a planned number of sessions are required which explore issues and how these are going to affect Jim once he is out in the community.

Case 4

1. Is this behaviour acceptable?

It may be acceptable when one understands and ascertains the reason for such behaviour. Whether it is acceptable after reflection becomes a matter of personal opinion, and as a consequence the extent to which the behaviour is tolerated. Whatever the response, it is important to consider that the behaviour may be related to the cerebral vascular accident. Often, people suffering from a stroke will exhibit inappropriate behaviour, mood swings and emotional outbursts. Those experienced in nursing stroke patients will see it for what it is – part of the condition.

2. What should be done about Percy's behaviour?

Nurses need an awareness of the possible reasons for this behaviour, and should understand that it may be related to his condition rather than character. This is an important issue; relating behaviour to personality instead of illness has a direct effect on patterns of care. Labelling can become an easy option: 'Dirty old man – you want to watch him.' 'Needs a cold shower, if you ask me.' Such remarks are a short step away from reality. The patient should be told in no uncertain terms that the behaviour is not appreciated, a remark that will need continued expression.

Case 5

1. Can the reduced sexual activity be attributed to the pain from the arthritis?

Yes and no. Remember, Mrs Lewis is at the peak of available treatments. Such treatments may include drugs which adversely affect sexual activity. Nonsteroidal anti-inflammatory drugs tend to cause indigestion and abdominal pain which, if persistent, can cause depression and apathy. Indomethacin causes the side-effects of headaches and drowsiness. Corticosteroids can also affect sexual drive. A reappraisal of drug treatment may have some bearing on reduced sexual activity.

2. How can Mary and her husband be helped?

The mainstay advice is 'if it feels good do it'. If whatever activity gives pleasure to both parties, and it does not offend, then carry on; for example, mutual masturbation, the use of vibrators. It is a time to experiment with different positions for love-making, and with adjustments to medication so that pain relief occurs before and during intercourse. Such a scenario warrants a nurse or other health care professional to be comfortable with discussing sexual issues of an intimate nature. The degree of success in helping Mary and her husband will depend on the knowledge base and depth of relationship the carer has.

Case 6

1. Why is Alan behaving in this way?

He is rebelling against the condition because of its interference with his lifestyle. He may see the procedures of giving injections and monitoring his diet at totally alien to his nature. The relationship with his mother may have altered as a result of his getting diabetes. His over-protective mother may remind Alan of his younger years. When he compares such behaviours with his peer group there may be wide discrepancies, which cause concern.

2. Could he have been treated differently?

It is easy to say yes at this point, because the whole story is available. However, in the 'real world' it is easy to see how the concept of sexuality may not have occurred to those looking after Alan. The mere clinical nature and manifestation of diabetes directs energies towards physical and physiological care. Such channelling could be to the detriment of psychological care, and in particular sexuality. Considering how Alan's sexuality might be compromised by the condition could have changed the pattern of care.

Case 7

1. Why did some of the nurses behave the way they did?

Unfortunately, there is evidence to suggest that doctors and nurses are intolerant of homosexuality, which has a direct effect on patient care (Kuczynski, 1980; Webb 1988), and that such attitudes are linked to actual behaviour (Webb and Askham, 1987).

From this it is easy to suggest that this case is not an isolated incident. The nurses in the scenario were acting upon, and making value judgements about, the behaviour and lifestyle of Mike. Such behaviour is born out of ignorance and fear about homosexuality. In order to be non-judgemental, nurses have to recognize and come to terms with their own feelings and attitudes towards issues such as homosexuality. For some this will be a taxing activity. However, raising awareness about sexual issues does affect the comfort level of nurses when they have to deal with sexuality in the nursing situation.

2. Is this a true representation of how gay people are cared for?

There is mounting evidence to suggest that gay people are being discriminated against in the health care setting (Jones, 1984; Jones, 1988). With the initial media coverage of HIV and AIDS and the strong homosexual connection, many nurses' attitudes and knowledge have been strongly influenced. The association between AIDS and homosexuality is inescapable.

> *For the first few years of the epidemic in the West it was seen as a gay disease.*
>
> Bancroft, 1989 (p. 326)

Case 8

1. Do you think the nurse covered the questions adequately?

Basically, the nurse did not answer the question, 'These tablets I'm taking – they're all right, I mean no side-effects or anything?' What the nurse discussed was what the tablets did, and not the side-effects. The hidden agenda here could have been an enquiry about how the tablets might affect sexual function. It is known that some anti-hypertensive drugs (particularly propranolol) can affect libido and lead to impotence.

2. Was there a deeper issue which was either unidentfied or avoided by the nurse?

The nurse did not pick up the cues, and was not specific enough in answering the question. What does 'everything in moderation' really mean? What was needed was a planned and specific breakdown of activities. In relation to sexuality, Ken was possibly searching for answers to questions about when he could resume sexual activity. Will he still be able to perform as before?

There is considerable evidence to suggest that there is a decline in sexual activity following a heart attack, with accompanying erectile problems (Bloch, Maeder and Harssly, 1975). A decline in sexual activity can have physical and psychological ramifications, it may also put strain on a relationship. The resumption of sexual activity should be allied to other forms of physical activity. This usually means a gradual progression, for example, climbing a flight of stairs, or taking a short walk. These activities are then increased, in the absence of any angina. It may be helpful to masturbate alone in order to test the consequence of the activity. The resumption of sexual activity should be titrated with the physical activity. The climbing of two flights of stairs (moderate exercise) is equivalent to sexual intercourse so long as it is non-vigorous. Where possible, all of these points should be discussed with the patient and his/her partner (Weinstein and Como, 1980).

Case 9

1. How should the situation be handled?

It is important in this situation to have some expertise or at least awareness of counselling skills, and possible treatments (see Chapter 6 for a discussion on skills). The counsellor should feel relaxed and confident in answering sexual issues. There should also be sufficient knowledge about human sexuality so that advice can be given confidently. Background information is required on the extent and nature of the problem (present scenario), together with desired outcome (preferred scenario).

The handling and process of the situation may include one or a collection of the following.

1. Supplying accurate information about the prognosis and behaviour (for example, as Jean's condition progresses how will it affect her sexual appetite? Will she still have the same desire for sex? Are other positions possible for sexual intercourse, and so on).
2. Giving specific advice. In this area advice is given about differing sexual techniques: self-stimulation, mutual masturbation and experimenting with different positions during sexual intercourse, for example. Other advice includes improving on communication, and tender expressions coupled with non-threatening touching and caressing ('sensate focus', Masters and Johnson, 1966).
3. Extending communication. Discussion about sexual activity should involve both parties. The appropriateness and effectiveness

of this will depend on the tripartite relationship, that is, husband, wife, counsellor. The prime objective here should be the development and cultivation of a secure emotional relationship.

Case 10

1. What may be the reasons for John's embarrassment?

He may find it difficult talking to another man about this aspect of his relationship. He may feel that the nurse will be judgemental about him and the problem. He may never have talked about personal sexual issues before. He may feel that he is less of a man for having this problem.

2. What may be an appropriate response to John's disclosure of the problems?

The nurse will need to take the problem seriously and convey a non-judgemental attitude. It is important to encourage him to provide clear information about the problems, while at the same time not pressurizing him to disclose more than he feels comfortable with. If John says that he has a specific problem with being able to have or maintain an erection, it would be appropriate to tell him that the GP will probably wish to ensure that there is no physical reason for this. It may not be appropriate to concentrate on the sexual problem to the exclusion of the original presenting problems.

3. How may John's situation have caused or contributed to his sexual problem?

Stress caused by his job and the uncertainty about his future may be a direct cause of his diminished sexual interest. Lying in bed and feeling anxious about his situation may well have been sufficient to affect his interest in sexual activity. This can become a vicious circle, as he may start to worry about his lack of interest. The couple's normal social interaction may have been altered by his increased workload. This may have resulted in their usual patterns of intimate behaviour being disrupted. One or both may have been affected by this, and their normal emotional or sexual feelings and behaviour may be altered as a result. There may be no connection between the job situation and his sexual problem; there may be other, as yet undisclosed, factors.

4. What would the CPN need to clarify with John during this session?

The facts, and how John feels about the problem. The nurse will need to obtain and clarify the history of the sexual problem. As this is the second session, the nurse should have general background information about the presenting problems and John's personal history. The disclosure of the sexual problem needs to be addressed in the context of the marital relationship and information obtained about this. Has the sexual problem caused other problems? John's understanding and beliefs about the problem need to be clarified. What, if anything, has either he or his wife attempted to do about this problem? Also, what is he willing to consider as help, for example, would he agree to his wife being seen?

5. What issues may the CPN need to consider before the next session?

His own skill and knowledge level. Is he equipped to provide the help that John may require? In discussion with the GP, they need to decide if more specialist help is required. If it is, then the effect on John must be considered. Will he want to start again with another person? If the CPN is continuing, does he feel comfortable in dealing with these problems? He needs to consider what approach to take with John in negotiating the direction and content of the work. Consideration needs to be given to seeing other family members, and also when and how to talk with John about this.

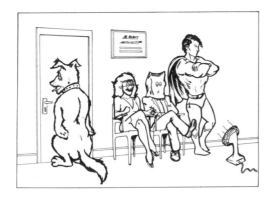

REFERENCES

Bancroft, J. (1989) *Human Sexuality and Its Problems*, 2nd edn, Churchill Livingstone, London.

Bloch, A., Maeder, J.P. and Harssly, J.C. (1975) Sexual problems after myocardial infarction. *American Heart Journal*, **90**, 536-7.

Hogan, R. (1980) *Human Sexuality. A Nursing Perspective*, Appleton-Century-Crofts, New York.

Jones, A. (1988) Nothing gay about bereavement. *Nursing Times*, **84**(23), 55-7.

Jones, R. (1984) With respect to lesbians. *Nursing Times*, **5**(18) 48-9.

Kuczynski, H.J. (1980) Nursing and medical students' sexual attitudes and knowledge: curriculum implications. *JOGN Nursing*, **11-12**, 339-42.

Masters, W.H. and Johnson, V.E. (1966) *Human Sexual Response*, Little, Brown, Boston.

Waterhouse, J. and Metcalfe, M. (1991) Attitudes towards nurses discussing sexual concerns with patients. *Journal of Advanced Nursing*, **16**, 1048-54.

Webb, C. (1988) A study of nurses' knowledge and attitudes about sexuality in health care. *International Journal of Nursing Studies*, **25**(3), 235-44.

Webb, C. and Askham, J. (1987) Nurses' knowledge and attitudes about sexuality in health care - a review of the literature. *Nurse Education Today*, **7**, 75-87.

Weinstein, S.A. and Como, J. (1980) The relationship between knowledge and anxiety about post-coronary sexual activity among wives of post-coronary males. *The Journal of Sex Research*, **16**(4), 316-24.

CHAPTER 9

Teaching sexuality

An old friend and mentor, Sir Clifford Norton, told me about sex education in Rugby before the First World War. The Headmaster, who must have been an enlightened man, summoned all the boys who had reached the age of puberty to his study and, after reassuring himself that the door was firmly secured, made the following brief announcement: 'If you touch it, it will fall off.'

Peter Ustinov (1992)

LEARNING OBJECTIVES

After reading this chapter you should be able to:

1. have an appreciation of how the subject of sex education has been treated in the past;
2. examine how sexuality might be taught in the future;
3. identify ways in which the subject of sexuality can be facilitated.

I'LL SHOW YOU MINE IF YOU SHOW ME YOURS

The opening remarks by Ustinov are to some extent an accurate picture of how the subject of sex education was treated by the Victorians. Indeed, people of that era would have considered themselves lucky if any mention of the subject was made at all. Greaves (1965) verifies that the first recorded formal endeavour at sex education was instigated by Dr Arnold, who coincidentally was the headmaster of Rugby School in 1828. It would appear that the basic aim and format of Arnold's sex education was to get his students to literally accept and adhere to certain passages in *The Bible*. For example:

> *Therefore shall a man leave his father and his mother, and shall cleave unto his wife: and they shall be one flesh. And they were both naked, the man and his wife, and were not ashamed.*

Genesis, 2, 24–25

The verse illustrates the importance of leaving the family home, marrying and procreating. Once in such a relationship, which should be ever-lasting, neither of the two shall stray.

> *It is good for a man not to touch a woman. Nevertheless, to avoid fornication, let every man have his own wife, and let every woman have her own husband. Let the husband render unto the wife due benevolence: and likewise also the wife unto the husband. The wife hath not power of her own body, but the husband: and likewise also the husband hath not power of his own body, but the wife.*
>
> Corinthians, 7, 1–5

The essence of this verse is the sanctity of marriage, the importance of fidelity, and the respect and control married couples should have over their own feelings. This shows that part, if not all, of the aspects of sex education at that time were about the avoidance of or abstention from any sexual activity outside wedlock. Those who did so indulge would encounter the consequences of their 'self-abuse'; for example, masturbation and the resulting physical and mental problems that were thought to ensue. It is clear that many of the early documents on sex education concentrated on instilling a correct moral code and decent standards of behaviour, usually decided by the church.

Trial and error

Humphries (1988) in his book (and television series by the same name), *A Secret World of Sex*, explored how sex education was treated in Victorian and Edwardian times. There was no overt sex education programme; most understanding about sexuality was by trial and error or gleaned from advice, which was not always correct and usually handed down to the younger generation from older brothers and sisters. Spying on courting couples or exploring each others' bodies was another method of attempting to understand this unmentionable subject. In one account in Humphries' book, this aspect of discovery is graphically explained.

> *We used to spy through a hedge on this couple who went over the recreation ground and did it. Well, you had to learn something by looking at something like that. Then we used to go out in the country and spot courting couples and see what they were getting up to. Sometimes the bloke would come over shaking his fist, saying 'Clear off you little swines!' We were only trying to learn something, weren't we? But you couldn't learn much because they all had their clobber on; they were muffed up to the eyeballs. We used to pick up a lot from the older boys. Once*

I was in chapel and a boy showed us all a contraceptive in a tin. He said he was using it on his girlfriend and was very proud of himself. Then there was this local girl; she used to take us out in the fields away from all the houses and display her wares to us. She'd take her clothes off and sort of put on a show. She was very proud of her body and we thought she was being very kind to let us look and have a feel. Because to us it was the eighth wonder of the world.

(page 35)

The level of understanding on sexual matters was different in the two social class extremes. The lower class children were better informed than upper class children. Independence from adult control is seen as the main cause of this discrepancy. Street gangs were a feature of the lower class way of life. This allowed for freedom, experimentation and exploration on each other; group masturbation and fondling of genitals was widely practised. Groups of young boys would hang around street corners flirting with the neighbourhood girls.

As a consequence of all this secrecy about sex and the sexual act, there were considerable misunderstandings. Some commonly held beliefs of the time were: that girls could get pregnant by sitting on lavatory seats after boys, or by kissing or even by touching a boy when menstruating. Sexual intercourse was considered safe if it was done standing up – 'because sperm can't travel upwards'!

As a result of this lack of informed sex instruction, most people had no knowledge about conception or childbirth. To some it would seem genuinely believable that babies were found under gooseberry bushes, or were brought by storks, or in the black bag doctors carried around. This ignorance lead to many women facing pregnancy and childbirth having no idea about what was taking place inside their own bodies, let alone what was going to happen to their bodies during childbirth and the period thereafter.

There are a number of reasons suggested for such ignorance. First, it may have been an attempt by parents to keep control over their sexually developing children, and to continue the guilt ridden Victorian attitudes of sexuality handed down by their parents. Second, it could have been that parents themselves were anxious and confused about their own sexuality. As a result, they refused to broach the subject with their developing children. Or that they felt ill-equipped to teach the subject and considered it the domain of others such as the church or school.

First formal teachings

One of the first major experimental studies involving sex education was carried out by Tucker and Prout in 1937. The survey examined seven Welsh education authorities. The results of the survey concluded that parents believed sex education to be 'acceptable and necessary'. When asked who should be responsible for this sex education they found: the children's fathers thought that sex education should be the mothers' domain, while mothers of the children thought that teachers should be responsible. To complete the confusion, the majority (94%) of teachers wanted the teaching to be done by specialists outside the profession. This chaotic state of affairs remained until 1943 when the Board of Education issued a directive stating that sex education was in the province of the teaching profession. This was possibly one of the most significant steps in achieving official recognition for the formal teaching of sex education.

In the unpublished Mass Observation survey of 1949 it was found that only 11% of the sample received any sex instruction from their mothers, while 6% received advice from their fathers. Daughters would receive information about sex in preference to sons, with the information usually given by the mother. Such information would usually revolve around advice about how to avoid sex, rather than any discussion about its associated feelings and desires. The survey also found that the great majority of those questioned said they had learned most about sex from workmates and friends.

The timing of such discussions for girls seemed to occur around the start of menstruation. Even the very normal act of menstruating was laden with secrecy, shame, fear and guilt. There seem to be some deep-rooted reasons for such feelings. It is suggested that the centuries-old religious belief was that the act of menstruation was part of God's curse for the sin of Eve. The phrase 'the curse' is still used by women today to describe menstruation. Or as one woman described it, 'No-one told me anything; when my periods started at 11 I thought I was bleeding to death' (Kilroy-Silk, 1992).

Might these social and psychological events affect in some way the physical aspects of sexuality? The age at which menstruation starts has slowly gone down. For Edwardian girls the average age at menarche was 15 years. By the 1960s it had reduced to 13. This phenomenon is not restricted to girls; boys, too, seem to be experiencing an early start to secondary sexual characteristics. In the early eighteenth century, young boys' voices dropped at a mean age of 17½, but they now drop at 13½ (Roche, 1979). This means that they have the potential for fertility two years earlier than their counterparts in the 1700s. Yet in neither girls nor boys is the capacity for reasoning, anticipation and planning fully developed until the age of 14 or 15. All this means that sexual maturity is occurring earlier than in past generations, while the capacity for predicting and coming to terms with the consequences of sexual activity is not (Tanner, 1968). Perhaps this is a noteworthy gap for sex education to fill? A gap that means a movement from the old idea that sex education is about sexual organs and their functions. It means encompassing the whole nature of sexuality itself – how men see the world, how women see the world. It is also about communicating needs, desires, feelings, behaviour, hopes and aspirations for the future, even to its most basic level of maintenance of the species.

Of course, the link suggested above, that social and psychological aspects of sexuality might have a physical consequence, is yet unproven, and so at the moment remains pure conjecture.

Teenage births and abortions

The effect of this early sexual development and resulting activity can be seen in the figures for births and abortions in teenage girls. In 1969 there were 6.8 births per 1000 among 16-year-olds in Britain. However, in 1986 the rate had risen to 8.7 per 1000 (Frater, 1986). In 1988, 3568 legal abortions were performed among under 16-year-olds, and 37 928 among 16 to 19-year-olds in England and Wales (OPCS Monitor, 1989).

A way out of this increase in teenage pregnancies is education about sex. 'Sex education should start at five, say MPs.' This remark prompted a headline in *The Independent* newspaper on 7 November 1991, and was made by a committee of MPs who make up the Parliamentary Health Select Committee. It was their response to stemming the tide of unplanned pregnancy. They suggested that sex education should be included in the National Curriculum for pupils aged five to 16. The committee went on to say that every school should have a specialist teacher with training in sex education. Other elements to be added to the curriculum were information on parenthood, contraceptive advice, and the nature and form of human relationships.

When these sentiments (as positive as they are) are seen within the school setting and the evidence available to date about teacher attitudes and desire to teach sex education, there is indeed an obvious mismatch. It would appear that work needs to be done on training and developing teachers for this role before improvements can be seen in the lifestyles of teenagers.

Activity 1: The birds and the bees

This activity asks you to explore how and by what means you learned about sex. Take a moment to discover your answers to the following questions (knowledge could also mean informa-tion):

1. How did you receive your knowledge about sex? (e.g. books, parents, friends, media, etc)
2. Where did you receive your knowledge about sex?
3. From whom did you receive your knowledge about sex?
4. Did you have sex education in school? If yes, how were the sessions handled? And in what subject was it taught?
5. Should sex education be different for men and women? (If 'yes' what would the differences be?)

Facilitator's notes (time allowance 1.5–2 hours):

Students could perform the activity in pairs or groups, with each group taking a particular question and then reporting back on the discussion to the whole group. The facilitator then co-ordinates the feedback, and identifies themes and areas of misunderstanding. The generation of uncertainty could form the basis for further work with the group, and as such provide areas of study. This activity could highlight weak areas in basic anatomy, physiology and reproduction. In so doing, it may indicate a need for remedial work before moving on.

Variations of the activity could include students taking the questions and using them as a structured interview guide. This guide could then be used to ask questions of people from a different generation to the student, i.e. parents, grandparents or even younger children. Care is required in regard to the latter point, with appropriate approval being sought. The information, once generated, will need to be displayed by appropriate means.

The treatment of sexuality by the Victorians is in stark contrast to today's treatment of the subject. Sex has become one of the most topical subjects of modern times. The Victorians pretended it did not exist; today's society seems to imagine that nothing else does. A casual look at any number of the weekly or monthly women's magazines that proliferate today will show the subject of sex and sexuality appearing repeatedly. The increase in men's magazines and their contents also highlights sexual issues. It would appear that daily newspapers, particularly tabloids, have also identified that sex can sell as many (if not more) copies than hard factual news. The 'page three girl' is an obvious case in point (*Daily Mail*, 1991; *Daily Express*, 1991; *Today Newspaper*, 1993).

Sex and sexuality are no respecters of class or position in society when it comes to news items; the exposure of the Royal family and their clandestine exploits is testimony to this. An increasing number of records made today for the 'pop' market have some reference to sex or sexuality. Next time you visit a record store, take a few minutes to look at the listing of the charts and see how many relate to or have lyrics about a sexual theme.

The media

McMahon (1990) examined the world-renowned women's magazine *Cosmopolitan* over a 12-year period from 1976 to 1988. Her study identified that the type of reader was young and married to a working class man. The majority of the women worked in clerical or public service facilities. This was in complete contrast to the image of the 'Cosmo girl' who was supposed to select her lover to match her moods and star sign.

The majority of articles in the magazine fell into six categories: relationships with men (77 articles); the lives of celebrities (51); explicit advice about sex (49); beauty, diet and health (34); psychological problems and advice (30); work and money (23). In selecting out these articles for further examination, McMahon found that sex was the key feature in all of them. Often the central foci were sexual problems, obsession or conflict. The articles on beauty, diet and health gave advice on how to create yourself into a desired object. Titles in issues have ranged from 'Sex with more than one partner' to 'Sadomasochistic sex'. The magazine has a circulation of over three million copies each month in the United States, with further editions being published in at least 12 foreign languages – sex is indeed big business.

It is important to point out at this stage that there is a difference between media sex and sex education. Just because there is a proliferation of sex in the media, it does not mean education is taking place as a consequence. In fact, the opposite could be said to be true. The exposure and availability of sexual literature is increasing. This rise in popularity appears to centre around material of a romantic nature (see Mills and Boon, Barbara Cartland or even the teenagers' magazine *Just Seventeen*).

Repercussions

This increased awareness appears to have had repercussions on the sexual activity of the younger age group in society. A Gallup poll published in September 1989 claimed that one in seven women aged under 25 had lost their virginity before leaving school, while one in eight men had had sexual experiences before the age of 16. In contrast, three quarters of women now aged over 44 had not yet had their first sexual encounter at the age of 20 (Hadfield, 1989).

More recent research from the study carried out by Johnson, Wadsworth, Wellings *et al.* (1992) between May 1990 and December 1991 among 18 876 men and women aged between 16 and 59 in the UK, gives greater detail on sexual activity. In a lifetime, on average, men aged from 16 to 59 would have 9.9 partners. For women of the same age range the average is 3.4, a factor that proves men are more sexually active than women over all age ranges. Early sexual experience may also have an effect on long-term sexual activity. Those who reported sexual intercourse before the age of 16 were most likely to report a greater number of partners. All of these sexual activity indicators have consequences on health care needs, in particular genitourinary medicine clinics and the services they provide in treatment, education and prevention. The generation of sexual lifestyles and its outcome is the main emphasis of the Johnson *et al.* study (1992).

In all of this apparent sin and debauchery there appears to be a saving grace – marriage, or more precisely, childbirth. Again from the Johnson *et al.* study (1992), women who reported having children in the last five years were significantly less likely to have more than one partner than those who did not have children. The same appears to be true for men, that is, those who had become fathers in the last five years were less likely to have extra-marital affairs than their contemporaries who had not had children. This can be applied to health care, and especially to women attending antenatal clinics, where anonymous prevalence testing for HIV may be taking place and who are more likely to be in monogamous relationships than other women of the same age group. This factor has obvious repercussions, which affect the interpretations of programmes set up to monitor HIV prevalence. It is obvious that making policy or judgements about the spread of the disease has major consequences when taking such data on face value.

The Conservative government under Margaret Thatcher had a notable driving force in promoting and valuing the concept of the family, and to some this may appear to be a return to Victorian values. However, in the light of the viewpoint expressed above, there may have been method in such promotion. A return to Victorian values is one mainly covert method society has used to control sexual behaviour. Are there others?

CONTROLLING ADOLESCENT SEXUALITY

The literature suggests that society has adopted three approaches in an effort to control what appears to be advancing adolescent sexuality. First, the Hindu and Moslem cultures, which advocate early marriage. In India 70% of the 15- to 19-year-olds are married; in Pakistan this figure is 73%. However, in Europe only 7% of this age group are married (Jones, Forrest and Goldman, 1985). Second is the idea of abstinence. Eastern cultures have this high on the list of methods of sexual control, as do African nations, who punish adolescent unmarried offenders, although those chastised are usually girls. Finally, the approach generally chosen by Western societies is sex education, contraception and abortion.

Reports which have examined comparisons internationally of pregnancy rates among 15- to 19-year-olds concluded that a high teenage pregnancy rate was not an inevitable consequence of liberal attitudes towards sex. Ashken and Soddy's study in 1980 points to the fact that it is the **type** of sex education that matters. If young people have an avenue for discussion about their sexual drives, either at home or in school, they are more likely to accept their own sexuality and take advice on family planning. This British study interviewed pregnant teenagers and concluded that more sex education was needed to reduce the rate of pregnancies. It went on to suggest that the target age should be 12- and 13-year-olds, and those in social classes four and five (Ashken and Soddy, 1980).

School sex education

But what kind and how much sex education takes place in our British state schools? It can be seen from the work above that there is some confusion about who is the best person to deliver information about sex. This confusion was a continuing theme throughout the 1940s and 1950s. There was a continuous stream of directives and guidelines issued by various bodies concerning the teaching of sex education in schools. If the government of that day (1940s and 1950s) had legislated in a positive manner towards sex education in schools, and had produced some indicators, the sporadic nature of sex instruction in schools today would have been improved immensely. The only piece of legislation to indicate the importance of sex education was the 1944 Butler Education Act. This Act made it the statutory obligation of the local education authorities (LEAs) to provide what the Act termed 'Health education for the spiritual, moral, mental and physical development of the community'.

The linking of sex education to other subjects such as health education seems to have continued through to today's curricula, as shall be seen later. It may be, though, that 'linking' is too soft a word – perhaps hidden away seems a much more appropriate marker. Sex education became part and parcel of subjects like biology, human biology, religious studies and even physical education. The rationale for the integration of sex education into so-called related topics may be indicated by the following quote:

> *To cut off sex education from other aspects of health education may mean*
> *surrounding it with not very desirable mystery.*
>   Ministry of Education (1957, page 44)

By the 1960s sex education was seen as the accepted responsibility of the LEAs, to be offered not as a subject in its own right but within other curriculum subjects. However, due to the autonomy of schools (an issue that is paramount today with some schools applying for self-governing status), nothing was done to ensure that **all** schoolchildren received an adequate sex education, a point that is still relevant today.

The result of this potential deficit of parity of learning about sex education has repercussions when starting to consider teaching nursing students about sexuality. It has even wider ramifications when one considers that, perhaps for the first time, young students may be coming into close contact with intimate body parts, and another person's feelings. It would be an agreeable state of affairs if students had the same grounding, skills and knowledge in sexuality as they had in, say, English, mathematics and biology.

New nursing students and their sex education

While researching for this book, a small-scale enquiry was conducted into discovering what formal sex education new students of nursing (three months and nine months into the course) could remember having in school. The methodology consisted of asking the students to jot down on a small card what formal sex education they had received in school. This was further qualified by asking them to consider their entire school career, that is, from infant school through to comprehensive or secondary education. The responses were anonymous, the only indicator was the person's age, which was used to collate the information. The following array of comments presents the findings from a total of 83 students.

Age 17–21 years (number of students, 27)

- 'Videos and books in junior school. Lady came into comprehensive school to talk about menstruation. Most was learned during discussions with friends, and in the playground.'
- 'None. (Few biology classes) we had a talk on periods.'
- 'Sex education was given in first year of comprehensive, one lesson per week for approximately six weeks, dealing with relationships etc, during the teens.'
- 'At school at the age of 11 we were told to ask our parents for permission to receive sex education; that was the worst part. When we had the information the teacher was more embarrassed than

us. In biology we learnt about frogs and worms from a red teacher.
As a Catholic school we were sent out in form 5 for natural family
planning. This was informative, but nobody tells you anything other
than the physical bits!'

- 'My fondest memories of school sex education was of being
marched in hoards of classes and crammed into our lecture theatre
and shown an extremely old film, vaguely covering points on
puberty, intercourse and pregnancy, birth etc. However, the lecture
theatre was so cramped with so many bodies in it, it was impossible for any of us to take the film seriously with so many nymphomaniac boys around.'

- 'Video – menstruation. Biology – reproduction in animals, plants
but **not humans**. General RE – AIDS and safer sex.

- 'Sex education was limited to a one-hour biology lecture and a 20
minute question time. Information was gained from peers and
naughty books.'

- 'We had a class of 30 pupils of mixed sex. Our sex education classes
were held on a Thursday afternoon by a male teacher. A very
relaxed atmosphere. The only lesson with full attendance.'

- 'Education started during second year at comprehensive. The
"Tampax" lady gave a talk about menstruation to the girls only.
Third year – given a video in lecture theatre: 'A month in the life
of sperm and egg' (biology GCSE). Fifth year – a talk from a
perverse PE teacher about not using crisp bags as condoms.'

Age 22–26 years (number of students, 18)

- 'Infants – no sex education, but told to use the bin in the toilet for
sanitary towels. In comprehensive about six lessons called 'PR'
(personal relationships), which explained menstruation, sexual
intercourse and having a baby. Not much contraceptive advice.'

- 'Reproduction lessons. Learned off parents. Off other people.'

- 'No formal sex education.'

- 'Primary schools – nil sex education. Secondary school, a 10 minute
talk on puberty, but nothing more than that.'

- 'We had two videos in the first year at the comprehensive, one
on female and one on male. During biology in the fourth year we
covered it through a textbook.

- 'Only in biology, but in no detail, nothing to do with facts of life
etc. Also because I went to a private all-male school, there was
absolutely nothing about the opposite sex. Also there was nothing
to do with sexually transmitted diseases. I read up on most of what
I now know.'

- 'We didn't have sex education classes; we just covered the
reproductive system in our biology lessons.'

Age 27–31 years (number of students, 12)

- 'Videos, formal teaching – biology masters, peer group. I received very little sex education, most of the information I gained was from my peers, books and magazines.'
- 'Basic female reproductive organ and male reproductive organ – no sex education as such.'
- '12 to 13 years old, not sure, one and half hours, outside speaker, lecture, some leaflets – included a talk on drink and drugs. I think it was a bit of a religious thing. Can't recall anything else.'
- 'Comedy cartoon film for whole class on all aspects of sex – e.g. male and female anatomy, sperm travel with cartoon character, Spike.'
- 'Very basic and formal. There was never any reference to loving and caring. It was delivered through lessons and videos in small classes.'

Age 32–36 years (number of students, 14)

- 'Infant–primary, none; information gained in playground. High school, some biology but most in break-times.'
- 'None. Perhaps if I had, I wouldn't have been a mother at such a young age.'
- 'Biology class – functional side; seminar type – functional side; small class chat, youth retreat – emotional side.'
- 'Playground talk, no formal at all.'
- 'Excellent, two years of full curriculum, lectures, films, seminars covering masturbation, oral sex, female and male orgasm, drugs and venereal diseases and contraception.'
- 'Video and slides on intercourse, fertilization, contraception etc. Teacher was very flustered and needed to loosen his shirt and tie when questioned.'

Age 37–40+ years (number of students, 12)

- 'No sex education at all. Pages on reproduction were cut out of old biology books.'
- 'Infant–primary – nil. Information from playground and family only. Secondary – formal at 16 years (three one-hour sessions, I think). Given by interested teachers. An enthusiastic effort but little new information, lacking in humour.'
- 'Talk from teacher on menstruation. Videos on reproduction and contraception. Peers.'
- 'Received physiology lessons on male and female reproduction. Very formal, never allowed to ask questions.'
- 'Sex education was non-existent. The only information I gained at school was given to me by other girls in the playground.'

The main observation on analysis of the above is the inconsistency in the teaching of basic knowledge and related areas of sexual matters. When looking at the students' comments over an age span, that is, what the 17-year-olds and 40+ year-old students are saying, the content and type of delivery seem to have a recurring theme, with the most common being the use of videos and films. However, overall, the comments are varied and mixed. This is not remarkable given that directives and guidelines on the subject were sketchy and lacking in any legislative power. The result of such mixed, and in some instances lack of, knowledge about sex and sexuality makes the teaching of it within the nursing context troublesome. Such disparity must be reflected in any teaching of the subject to nursing students. It would seem appropriate that to overcome such an unequal distribution of understanding, a considered and comprehensive curriculum model on sexuality should be implemented. The aspect of curriculum models and methods of teaching sexuality will be considered later. The discussion now returns to the aetiology of sex education within state schools.

INTEGRATED SEX EDUCATION

By the mid 1970s the idea of having sex education as an integral part of the school timetable was well established (Rea, 1974). The Department of Education and Science (DES) did give some guidelines regarding the content of sex education (1977), but, unfortunately, ideas about reducing inconsistency throughout the country were not discussed. Two controversial statements appear in this document (DES, 1977).

1. Allowing the head of schools discretionary powers as to the inclusion of birth control.
2. The decision about the appropriateness of including all the details on aspects of sexual intercourse.

The two points are interesting in that they raise the issues of morality and ethics behind the subject of sex education. There is the danger that the teaching and trend of sex education is fashioned around the sexual mores of the teacher, and not around the needs of the students, a factor that any teacher should consider fully before embarking on the teaching of a sex education programme.

Reflecting on the following questions may serve as an indicator of appropriateness to teach.

- 'Am I at ease with my own sexuality and therefore able to teach others?'
- 'Do I have a degree of knowledge about the anatomy and physiology of reproduction?'

- 'Do I understand others who may have differing views to my own?'
- 'Can I deal with the subject sensitively, respecting student autonomy?'
- 'Do I appreciate that lifestyles may be different from my own?'
- 'Can I facilitate an understanding about varying attitudes?'
- 'Do I understand, and am I able to facilitate an awareness in others, that sexual expressions may vary?'

If one reflects on the reports, directives and ideas in the last few years, they appear to be suggesting the following: (1) sex education should become part of various sections of the curriculum; (2) there is a need for special training for teachers; and (3) there is a need to involve parents in sex education, so it becomes a collaborative venture. It is interesting to speculate how these three points apply to the field of nurse education. Substituting patients for parents may provide a tripartite model under which sexuality may be considered in the nursing curriculum.

SEX EDUCATION IN THE 1980s AND 1990s

One of the major effects on sex education during this period has been the 1980 Education Act. The Act produced legislation which required LEAs to inform parents of the way and context in which sex education was to be provided (Hansard, 1980). The context in which sex education was taught was given considerable debate. Should it remain under the umbrella of health education or be integrated into the human and social development (pastoral) parts of the school curriculum? This argument continues to this day.

By 1984 there was still no uniform pattern in the teaching of sex education in UK schools (Family Planning Association, 1984). In a study carried out by Thomas in 1986, eight Welsh LEAs were asked for their policies, together with aims and objectives on sex education. In reply, none stated they had any form of policy, aims or objectives on sex education. In 1987 the DES outlined the clear responsibility of schools to ensure that 'pupils are adequately prepared for adult life' and stressed the importance of parental views in formulating a sex education policy. The DES went on to recommend presentation of the facts, which should include controversial issues, in an objective, balanced manner to encourage the development of informed, reasoned and responsible attitudes. This was hoped to encourage both sexes to behave in a responsible manner where sexual matters were concerned.

This is the first record of directives indicating the importance of a collaborative approach. The significance of this later aspect has been indicated in another study. Jackson (1989) looked at the content and attitudes of sex education in 17 secondary schools in the Cheshire area. The results and conclusion showed that a variety of programmes took place. Those teachers involved did not feel comfortable nor adequately prepared to teach what they considered to be a difficult subject. There were, however, a number of strengths: parents liked to be involved in discussing sex education; the pastoral syllabus was followed up by the form tutors, thus ensuring continuity; and student-led sex education programmes progressed to personal and social developments.

Scott and Thomson (1992) describe the result of a survey carried out by the Sex Education Forum in 1991. The Sex Education Forum was formed in 1987 as a collection of interested parties (24) involved in supporting and propagating sex education in schools. The Forum was supported by a grant from the DES which enabled it to produce a document on a framework for school sex education.

The fundamentals of the document spell out the importance of knowledge, skills, values and attitudes in sex education. The survey contended that sex education was being carried out in a confused, inconsistent manner – what the authors termed 'more a patchwork than a pattern'. The teachers questioned found that uncertainty and embarrassment were the prime problems (68%). Factors affecting this could be traced to the Gillick ruling of 1986, together with Section 28 of the Local Government Act (1988). Both of these may have affected teachers' willingness to become involved in discussing concepts of a potentially contentious nature. Time and space within a busy curriculum were other factors affecting the implementation of any sex education programmes.

The effect of AIDS

One of the great outside forces of the late 1980s which has affected health education in schools is the condition AIDS. The emergence of this disease has had repercussions on the format and content of health education in schools, and of course its related sexual connotations (Bury, 1991). Could the same be said of sex education in schools of nursing? The DES (1986) produced a booklet called, *Children at School and Problems Related to AIDS*. If we were to play devil's advocate for a moment, we might consider that perhaps something positive has come out of the disease AIDS in respect of raising awareness and the importance of sexuality. This may be evidenced by the DES booklet and its note:

Schools should see it part of their task, in the context of personal and social education, to consider with pupils some of the broader questions

associated with the transmission of infection, including the health risks
of promiscuous sexual behaviour, whether heterosexual or homosexual.

DES (1986, p. 7)

There are a number of assumptions on the part of the DES. First, that the above is possible because each student receives a form of health education and, second, that teachers are prepared and able (which is not one and the same thing) to discuss promiscuous sexual behaviour and homosexuality. The DES appears to labour under the mis-apprehension that the directives and guidelines will be carried out when it is obvious that the human machinery is not in place.

EMERGENCE OF THE NATIONAL CURRICULUM

September 1986 heralded the Education Act. In section 18, paragraph 2, it required all county-controlled and maintained special schools:

1. to consider separately (while having regard to the local education authority's statement under section 17 of this Act [on their policy in relation to the secular curriculum in maintained schools]) the question whether sex education should form part of the secular curriculum for the school;
2. to make and keep up to date a separate written statement:
    (a) of their policy with regard to the content and organization of the relevant part of the curriculum;
    (b) or where they conclude that sex education should not form part of the secular curriculum, of that conclusion.

This state of affairs has been further refined with the Education Reform Act of 1988 and the emergence of the National Curriculum Council making the statutory orders and recommendations on curricula content. Within the orders of the National Curriculum there are four key stages which spell out both the programme of study and the attainments to be reached for each of the subjects within the National Curriculum (National Curriculum Council, 1991). Health education, which is cross-curricula theme number five, contains six areas: (1) substance use and misuse; (2) sex education; (3) family life education; (4) safety; (5) health-related exercise; and (6) food and nutrition. Again, each of the key stages has a programme of study and attainment targets. For example, the programme of study in key stage one (primary school) involves pupils finding out about themselves and their development: how they grow, feed, move and use their senses, and information is given about the stages of human development.

Attainment targets

The attainment targets for each of the four key stages cover a range of issues. For example, in key stage one (primary school) attainment targets are: (1) to know that humans develop at different rates; (2) to be able to name parts of the body, including the reproductive system, and understand the concept of male and female; (3) to know about personal safety, and that there are differences between good and bad touches; (4) to appreciate ways in which people live together.

When pupils reach higher secondary education (fourth and fifth forms) the programme of study directs pupils to extend their study of the major organs, and organ systems and life processes. Attainment targets are: (1) to understand aspects of Britain's legislation relating to sexual behaviour; (2) to understand the biological aspects of reproduction; (3) to consider various aspects of family planning; (4) to recognize and be able to discuss sensitive issues such as conception, HIV/AIDS and abortion within a framework which considers and respects attitudes, values, beliefs and morality; (5) to be aware of preventive health care; (6) to be aware that statutory and voluntary organizations exist to support human relationships.

Never before has the aspect of sex education, and for that matter health education, been so clearly mapped out. The literature and guidance being produced by the National Curriculum Council is giving teachers a clear message about the content and style of teaching. But is all this information and fine talk making a difference to the teachers and then ultimately the pupils? Voices can be heard suggesting that all is not well with sex education in schools. A committee chaired by Derek Dean of the professional Nursing, Midwifery and Health Visiting Association in England, warns that at least 50% of schools do not encourage sex education and discussion on related issues. In a letter to Mr Calman, Chief Medical Officer at the Department of Health, he says, 'If we are to achieve a greater degree of sexual health among the population, it is imperative that young people are given an early introduction and encouraged to discuss and explore sexuality in a secure setting with appropriate guidance' (*Nursing Times*, 1993).

When this response is seen within the context of the White Paper, *The Health of the Nation* (1992), which set a target for the number of teenage pregnancies to be halved by the year 2000, it presents an interesting state of affairs. It would seem obvious that some form of sex education and advice needs to be given to young people. Yet the subject of sex education in schools is still dogged by attitudes which are reminiscent of the Victorian era. This confusion about sex education within the state system has to be considered when educators have to develop nursing curricula. It is obvious that students of nursing will have a varied, and in some case non-existent, understanding of sexuality.

There needs to be a liberation of ideas and values within the state education system allowing teachers to seek the training, development and support they need in order to carry out this immensely important activity.

The following activity may uncover some of the aspects discussed above. It also highlights some of the problems which may be encountered in attempting to develop a sex education programme.

Activity 2: What shall we tell the kids?

This activity asks you to consider putting together a sex education session for different groups of people. When doing so, consider the following areas:

1. Who would teach the session?
2. How long should the session run for?
3. Outline the content of the session.
4. By what method should the session be taught?

Try designing a session for the following groups:

- Infant school children (4 to 6 years).
- Junior school children (7 to 11 years).
- Secondary school children (12 to 17 years).
- College students (17 to 21 years).
- Adults (21 years plus).

Facilitator's notes (time allowance, arbitrary):

Students can be split into smaller groups to draw up their various plans. After a stated time the facilitator invites the groups back to discuss their suggestions.

A variation could be to ask students to discover what sex education takes place for each of the identified groups. The areas 1 to 4 above then form a framework for structuring the findings, or an interview guide.

THE TEACHING OF SEXUALITY IN NURSING

It has been seen that the content of sex education in schools is inconsistent. Some schools have an identified programme of instruction, while for others it is just a hit-and-miss affair.

But how has the subject of sexuality been treated in nursing? Has this disparity of knowledge of sexual matters in nursing students been identified, and appropriate syllabus changes made? The short answer to this is 'no'. The reasons for this could relate back to the roots of nursing itself. It should be remembered that nursing was originally performed by such people as monks and nuns, and later by people like Florence Nightingale and women from higher social classes, not exactly the ideal people to contemplate discussing sexuality and patient care.

Compounding the problem were the morals and values of the time. Florence Nightingale believed that nurses should promote the image of a 'good wife', and be exemplary ladies of the time. Such ingredients are hardly a recipe for debate on what would appear to them an odious and inconceivable subject.

For a considerable time, the ethos of nursing has had to deal with (and will continue to deal with) the image and sentiments left by such people as Florence Nightingale, an image that many people, including the general public, still believe exists. There appears to be a commonly held belief that to nurse one has to be dedicated, desire a vocation, and have unquestioning dutiful service to the patient, as well as being a hand maiden to the doctor.

What is being hinted at here is that to some extent the image of the profession will dictate how and what the profession, and the people within that profession, should and should not do (Chapman, 1977; Etzioni, 1969). If nurses are to discuss and believe that concepts such as sexuality and expressing sexuality are important aspects of patient care (Roper, Logan and Tierney, 1980), then it calls for them to be proactive, and move it up the nursing agenda. In so doing they identify what society wants from its nurses and from nursing. But before going headlong into this debate, perhaps a note of caution needs to be made and a few questions asked. Does society want nurses to discuss and instigate care for concepts such as sexuality? To what extent do nurses become proactive, or should they be reactive? There are no easy answers to these questions, as we have seen from discussions in Chapter 3. But if teachers of nursing are to teach the subject of sexuality, and consider it an essential aspect of care, then they should be aware of the ramifications, some of which have been highlighted in Chapter 3.

However, the mark of a profession is that it works from a body of knowledge. The level of knowledge at present on how patients' sexuality is cared for is still growing. Such development should be encouraged and built upon, as there is still a great deal to learn about this fascinating subject. A deeper understanding of subjects like sexuality should be synonymous with improvement in patterns of care.

Recent work has made nurses aware of sexual problems, but these are cases where the sexual organ is involved and so initial awareness is usually raised in any case (Webb and Wilson-Barnett, 1983). Sexuality is an all-embracing aspect of being human, and so affects people all of the time, whether they are ill or well. Therefore, if a patient is admitted for a simple appendicectomy need nurses consider the effect on his/her sexuality, when compared to a patient having a hysterectomy? Many nurses do not engage either cognitively or linguistically with the concept of sexuality and the patient (Payne, 1976; Quinn-Krach and Van Hoozer, 1988; Webb, 1987). Whether this is due to a weakness in nurse education programmes or nurses' own sensitivity to the subject is questionable. There is evidence for both cases (Thomas, 1990; Waterhouse and Metcalfe, 1991; Webb, 1985).

The 'taboo family'

To some extent sexuality may have a similar developmental history to a close cousin of the 'taboo family' – death. Twenty or more years ago death was a little talked about subject, yet today it is well integrated into the nursing curriculum, even to the extent of having separate courses ('Death and dying' post-registration module). Will the same be said of sexuality? Is, or should, sexuality be taught across the curriculum? Chapter 1 explains how all-invasive the subject is; it crops up in many if not all subject areas. There is a parallel with this idea within the state school system, as has been seen. The problem of the cross-curricula method is that it becomes difficult to monitor and evaluate progress. One should remember also that not all teachers are comfortable with the subject, which could hinder its acknowledgement. An anecdotal account adequately demonstrates this last point. During an anatomy and physiology lecture on the male reproductive system, which was given by an experienced female teacher, a student asked what the function of the prostate gland was. The response from the teacher was, 'You're a man, you should know'! What the teacher was unable to discuss, despite her years of experience, was the role of the prostate in reproduction. The lack of knowledge on the student's part has repercussions in patient care, and the permissibility of raising sexual issues again with teaching staff. Of course, it is not fair to suggest that all teachers are prudes.

Meredith (1984), in an article about running a workshop for teachers on the subject of sexuality, makes a number of observations. Some teachers fear being labelled, for example, 'If I talk about sex to the students they might think I enjoy it.' Others think teaching about sexuality may reflect their own lifestyle: 'I have not had a satisfactory sexual relationship for some time and feel uncomfortable talking about female and male genitals.' While some felt they lacked the skills and confidence: 'I don't know how to describe some of the concepts and feel the students will see me as old-fashioned and silly.'

What these sentiments identify is the need for some form of self-appraisal before going headlong into teaching the subject matter. To some extent the teaching and learning of sexuality is as fulfilling for the teacher as it is for students. In achieving this, the teacher, or rather facilitator, has to be more involved with the participants so that a degree of acceptance and honesty is attained. Later on in this chapter the aspect of the teacher's role will be given more attention, when a proposed series of teaching sessions is outlined.

Before moving on to examine in more detail how the subject of sexuality has been treated in schools of nursing and in the literature, the following activity should be tried. Its purpose is to instigate interest. For some it will stir up memories of good and bad education and good and bad clinical practice.

Activity 3: No sex please, we're nurses

This activity asks you to think about the subject of sexuality during your nurse training/practice.

1. Was/is/should sexuality be taught as a separate subject, or a continual theme?
2. Did the subject of sexuality come up at all during your training? If it did, can you describe the circumstances?
3. Have you encountered problems concerning sexuality when working on the wards or community? If yes, can you describe the circumstances?
4. Have staff displayed differing views and attitudes about a patient's sexuality?
5. Have there been any occasions during clinical practice that patient care has been affected because of their sexuality?

Facilitator's notes (time allowance 1–2 hours):

The basic aim of this activity is to open up the awareness of students to the importance of sexuality in nursing care. It is usual for a considerable amount of anecdotal accounts to be generated. It is important that the session does not turn into a story-telling activity. Accounts that are discussed should have their problems and main points indicated. Where possible, solutions should be discussed and solutions found.

Variations of the activity could involve students role-playing a particular account they have discussed. A point of consideration with regard to roles may be made, in that students who are seen to hold strong ideas and attitudes about how a person should be handled, should attempt to play an opposing role. For example, if the scenario revolves around the treatment of a homosexual patient, and a student has a strong negative attitude about homosexuality, then she should be encouraged to adopt the role of the patient.

Care is needed not to force students into role-playing, and the necessary debriefing of students should be performed after the role play (Morry van Ments, 1983).

SEXUALITY IN NURSING TEXTS AND IN THE CURRICULUM

The earliest account of sexuality, or what might allude to sexuality, can be found in nursing texts of the 1960s and 1970s. A number of books were surveyed which revealed no direct reference to the subjects of sex or sexuality. Two examples of texts of the time were *The General Textbook of Nursing* (Pearce, 1960) and *Basic Nursing*, 3rd edition (Bendall and Raybould, 1970). The first book describes the physical aspects of a person's sexuality, which involves the care of the patient's genitalia in some way. There is no direct reference to sexuality in any psychological sense, nor in respect of being feminine or masculine. There are, however, some clues in the text that refer to how men and women were cared for differently. Bathing the patient is one such example.

The nurse will bathe a female patient, paying attention to the points described in giving a blanket bath. For a male patient, an attendant will be required unless the ward sister considers this unnecessary, in which case he bathes himself and, after he has returned to bed, the nurse ascertains that he is quite clean.

Pearce (1960, page 54)

Similarly, in Bendall and Raybould's book, some 10 years later, things still appear to be the same:

The patient is assisted from his bed to the bathroom, all toilet requisites being collected from his locker. Pyjamas are placed on the radiator to warm, and if necessary the patient is helped into the bath. Where a male patient needs assistance or supervision, it is customary for a male nurse or orderly to accompany him; in the case of female patients, the nurse will stay.

Bendall and Raybould (1970, page 45)

These two quotes divided by 10 years show amazing similarity, and are in stark contrast to today's practices. No material could be found that made reference to the psychological needs of male and female patients and their sexuality. These early days of nursing tended to concentrate on the very physical and practical aspects of care. A collection of the popular *Nurses Aid Series* were also examined for 'signs' of sexuality, but to no avail (Armstrong and Wakeley, 1959; Sayer and Semple, 1958).

The Americans, on the other hand, have been much more productive in terms of word and deed on the subject of sexuality. Lewis, a Chicago physician, was possibly the first person to attempt to put something into print about sexuality by attempting to discuss 'The hygiene of the sexual act' (Lewis, D. in Bullough and Seidl, 1987). The editors of the journal it was bound for – *The Journal of the American Medical Association* – refused to publish the article. They may have heeded the comments of a notorious gynaecologist of the time, Howard Kelly, who remarked 'discussion of the subject is attended with filth, and we besmirch ourselves by discussing it in public.' The publication of such an article would not be a problem today, considering the wealth of journals devoted to the subject of sexuality: *The Journal of Sex and Marital Therapy, The Journal of Sex Research, Sexuality and Disability, The Journal of Homosexuality, Archives of Sexual Behaviour, Medical Aspects of Sexuality.*

In the text of *American Nursing* the earliest account and excellent example of prudish behaviour is in Robb's book, *Nursing: Its Principles and Practice for Hospital and Private Use*, printed in 1907. Following on from the two British examples of bathing the patient, Robb's description refers to washing the surfaces between the thighs, and states that vaginal examinations were to be made 'under cover'.

So far, this enquiry has looked at the written word as evidence of how the subject of sexuality was treated, a somewhat covert stance. In an account of how male physicians treated female health problems, Waltley (1983) illustrates how women were treated differently purely on grounds of gender, or perhaps more precisely because they had a uterus. The uterus was seen as a 'link organ', in that it had control over other organs in the woman's body. It was excitable and so intimately connected to many nerves over the whole body that any upset would have far-reaching repercussions. It was as if the Almighty, in creating the female sex, had taken the uterus and built up a woman around it. Other writers have suggested that the uterus goes beyond pure physical control, but involves the intellect of the woman.

Galton in 1870 in his study of genius concluded from evidence which included the fact that the male brain was heavier than the female, that women had no mental resources for effective intellectual competition with men. This was graphically displayed in anatomical illustrations of women. The drawings showed women as having tiny heads, with an exaggerated pelvic width. This emphasized the supposed lower intelligence and the child-bearing roles women should occupy. Yet all was not gloom and doom for women; they were thought to have some redeeming qualities. They are elevators and civilizers of mankind, they nurture our young and are respecters and promoters of the arts, they are a moderating influence on the aggressive nature of man. Megis, a nineteenth century obstetrician, is reported as giving special lectures to his medical students on the attributes of women. From lecture notes he is recounted as saying: 'It is a woman's smile which makes man's achievements possible' (Donegan, 1975).

Present-day literature

As research for this chapter, a small-scale enquiry was carried out of present-day nursing literature and their sexual/sexuality content. The following identifies the popular journals, and the number of items written which contain a sexual/sexuality theme during 1982 to 1993 (total number, 64).

- *Nursing Times*   39 items
- *Journal of Advanced Nursing*   9   ''
- *International Journal of Nursing Studies*   2   ''
- *Nursing Research*   3   ''
- *Journal of Nursing Education*   11   ''

In just over nine years a total of 64 articles with a sexuality theme were written. It would be foolish to make sweeping comments about such a finding. They are presented here for the sake of interest, and possibly as a catalyst for discussion as to the possible reasons. When looking at books containing a sexuality theme, the Royal College of Nursing Library (the largest nursing library in Europe) was contacted and asked for a listing of books with sexuality in the title, together with their popularity of loan. In all, 66 titles were identified. The top three were: (1) Savage (1987), *Nurses, Gender and Sexuality*; (2) Hogan (1980), *Human Sexuality: A Nursing Perspective*; and (3) Llewellyn-Jones (1991), *Everyman*. These are also presented for speculative interest. It should also be remembered that just because a book is popular and is frequently out on loan does not mean it gets read. (Present book is, of course, an exception!)

There is then in nursing a smattering of literature on the subject of sexuality. Before entering the realms of ways of teaching the subject, its credibility as a subject should be established. In other words, why teach sexuality? To a certain extent this has been covered in Chapter 3 on sexuality and ethics – 'Is it any of our business?' What follows here is the 'framing' of the subject within a teaching

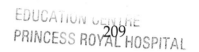
perspective. The bold type in the text that follows identifies the core themes within the teaching perspective and as such could be used as a main indicator in opening debate for initial sessions.

WHY TEACH SEXUALITY?

The principal aim of this section is to assist the nurse teacher in understanding methods, style and possible content of lessons on sexuality. However, it could be just as easily applied and used by the practising nurse as a simple teaching plan in the clinical setting, or as a self-taught programme of study. At its broadest remit the elements identified in the model could form the framework to a curriculum for a large course on sexuality.

As nursing moves towards a more holistic approach to patient care, there must be the general recognition that this totality of care takes into account the patient's sexuality. This is particularly the case if sexuality is understood to be concerned with all aspects of the individual, not just with the care of the genitalia. So the first premise for teaching the subject of sexuality could be identified as an **holistic approach to patient care**.

Sexuality encapsulates a wealth of emotions and experiences which makes it problematic to grasp and see the concept in its entirety. It affects our every-day life, whether we are aware of it or not. It is crucial that this is discussed and, where possible, parameters to the meaning of sexuality are recognized. In short, what is this subject called sexuality? What is it made up of? The second premise is: **concept clarification**.

The issue of sexuality could be evaded by teacher and student because, rightly or wrongly, they already know all about it. It is therefore assumed that, regardless of their age and experience in life, each nurse can deal confidently with their patients' sexuality because they understand and have come to terms with their own. Although life experiences may help a person to cope and come to terms with other people's sexuality (bearing in mind that coping and coming to terms is not one and the same thing), it is doubtful whether anyone is ever completely at ease with all forms of sexual expression. This then forms the third premise: **value clarification**.

Present-day expectations of the work patterns of nurses are quite high. The influx of ideas such as the nursing process, primary nursing, the name nurse and individualized holistic patient care have all played their part in increasing the quality of the nurse–patient relationship. This has crucial implications in the way nurses actually work and will be influenced by the patients' and nurses' personalities, past histories and the attitudes and work practices of the organization. This increase in the degree of intimacy in the nurse–patient relationship has a consequence when considering sexuality. It is important to remember that nurses do not cease to be human by virtue of wearing a uniform, although some may use it as a shield if the relationship gets out of control. Nurses are not disembodied workers without any self-awareness of what is happening around them. Yet they continue to cope with the remarkable and continued access they have to the bodies and emotions of their patients. There is, of course, an assumption to this last point of 'access to bodies and emotions'. Some nurses may not be comfortable with, nor see the necessity in 'getting too close' to the patient. As a consequence, their work patterns, style and depth of relationship will be different to those nurses who believe in a deeper, more committed patient contact.

Those nurses who attempt and achieve a degree of intimacy with their patients must be aware of the complexities and importance of such a relationship. Often the patient's private thoughts and feelings are reserved for, or even prohibited to, the patient's own partner. Such a relationship is not to be entered into lightly. It requires putting as much effort into the initiation and maintenance of the relationship, as it does in its eventual termination. When one marries these ideas to the subject of sexuality, with all its inherent delicate and private factors, it becomes even more obvious just how important it is that appropriate care is given.

There is evidence to suggest that nurses do not enter into or discuss the concept of sexuality because of the anxiety it produces in themselves as well as in patients (Kautz *et al.*, 1990; Miller, 1984). Entering into the patient's world, and being familiar with his or her feelings could be seen as a paradox of nursing. For some the sheer enjoyment of nursing is the development of and the involvement in the nurse–patient relationship, and yet it has the potential to be the most pernicious. The fourth premise is the **nurse–patient relationship**.

While engaged in the nurse–patient relationship, the nurse has to identify and help solve any problems the patient may have or may develop. In identifying and solving problems, a sound, up-to-date knowledge base of nursing is essential. The technology of medicine is increasingly dynamic both in its accomplishments and its mischief. This taxes the nurse's ability to be aware and informed of treatments and prognosis of the patients in their care. Treatments, whether medical, surgical, psychological or pharmacological, will affect the patient's sexuality to a greater or lesser extent. The fifth and final premise becomes **the impact of illness on sexuality**.

A suitable model

These five premises are not conclusive. Hopefully, what they will do is mark out a possible starting point, or framework, in which the teaching of sexuality could take place. The premises now need to be placed within a model in order to facilitate teaching. There appear to be three suitable models available for this purpose: (1) Burnard's (1990) simple curriculum model of aims and objectives, content, methods and evaluation; (2) Vincent's model (1968, in Walker, 1971) suggests a process model involving desensitization, sensitization and finally incorporation; and (3) Mandetta and Woods (1974) consider how certain aspects of sexuality affect the biological, psychological and social make-up of human beings.

It is not within the scope of this book to examine and apply all three curricula models and premises to the teaching of sexuality. However, it is important that one of the models is used as an example so that application can be demonstrated. The subsequent section will move through a proposed course on sexuality using the curriculum model of Vincent (1968). There is, however, an addition to the original framework, that is, the concept of identification. The rationale for this is that it would seem logical that anybody studying sexuality before desensitizing themselves to a given issue would need first to consider identifying the issue/s. In other words, you have to know what you are desensitizing yourself to.

TEACHING SESSIONS ON SEXUALITY

The role and function of the teacher

Before commencing any teaching session which has the potential to provoke anxieties for all concerned, the teacher has to ask and consider the answers to a number of questions. First, and most importantly, 'Am I comfortable with my role in teaching this subject matter?'

Because the subject matter can be sensitive and emotive, it is best tackled in a group setting (Koch, 1985; Ludlow and Bagwell, 1983; Meredith, 1984). It is within such a setting that students can express their fears and ideas, and examine their own and others' feelings about sexuality. One of the principal factors which will control the depth and effectiveness of the sessions is the idea of trust. Trust is not a concept that is declared, but it is a concept that has to be demonstrated to be meaningful. This means that the teacher will have to set the level and atmosphere of the discussion, usually by means of example, at least as a starting point.

The degree to which the teacher allows his or her own personal side to show through depends to a greater or lesser extent on the commitment to the subject, and experience in group work. It would be foolish to suggest that the teacher can become fully integrated into the group. The mere fact that he/she is a teacher, and as such represents authority, is inescapable. Where possible the teacher should explore this with the group. If this conflict of interests is opened up for discussion, it can go some way to demonstrating to the students the nature and role the teacher is taking. Of course, one must remember that the personality and character of the students involved is also a deciding factor on how well the group performs, but this is beyond the control of the teacher to some extent.

Group dynamics will always play a part in the life and productivity of the group and its generation of a learning environment. From experience, the degree of 'teacher exposure' is directly proportional to the depth and quality of the learning atmosphere and environment. It requires the teacher to adopt a different role than that of font of knowlege and deliverer of information. For the teacher who spends most of his or her time teaching by way of lectures or using a didactic format, it can be a terrifying idea to consider using a discussion or experiential learning group format. Thus the teacher must have a certain amount of self-awareness and confidence before contemplating teaching a sexuality programme.

In entering into the spirit of such a teaching method or style, it is important to identify that, primarily, you are an individual and next a teacher or nurse. As a teacher you must show your individuality, and this often takes the edge off the distinction between teacher and students. A suitable starting point to gauge your appropriateness to teach the subject of sexuality may be to consider your responses and feelings to the following activity.

Activity 4: Can I cope?

Consider your responses and feelings to the following points. You may like to share your findings with a colleague to see if opinions differ.

1. I am interested in the subject of sexuality because ...
2. It is important that students understand the subject of sexuality because ...
3. What will it *feel* like for me to talk about, and for people to ask me questions about, my own sexuality?
4. How would I respond if I found that the confidence of the group I was working with had been broken?
5. Will I be able to say, describe and explain sexually implicit words and meanings? (Look at the glossary of words in this book; try saying a couple of them out loud to yourself. What happens?)

6. Do I have the necessary interpersonal skills to teach this subject?
7. Am I comfortable with and able to discuss varying forms of sexual expression and behaviour?
8. Can I show an application of sexuality to nursing?

From your answers to Activity 4, together with the discussion on the role of the teacher in teaching sexuality, it becomes apparent that the term 'teacher' may be somewhat inappropriate. As has been highlighted, the emotive subject of sexuality is best discussed using a group setting. Doing group work demands a different set of characteristics and behaviours from the more popular didactic approach.

The term 'facilitator' would seem a more fitting description of the teacher role. The role and function of a facilitator in a sexuality programme should be outlined from the start. This initial outline will 'set the scene' for the process and will affect the working atmosphere of the group. The role of the facilitator may have to be outlined on more than one occasion. From experience it appears that teacher involvement with a group has to be spelt out; for as the group matures, the role of facilitator may become blurred. This blurring is to some extent a measure of the facilitator's ability to merge or become part of the group. The group may move on to directing itself (the members) to discussing various topics which are issues to different group members. Conversely, this may cause the group to lose direction and regulation. A method of testing and controlling this is to allow a member (or members) of the group to take up the role of facilitator, or lead. Such action may cause a halt in proceedings, with the question being asked, what is the subject matter? Member/s who act as facilitators for the group should physically take up the usual (teacher facilitator's) position in the circle. This gives the facilitator the advantage of observing the group from a different perspective. The change in setting is often all that is required to literally see the group and its members from a different angle. It also gives the facilitator time to rest.

Of course, the group has to have reached a stage of maturity and competence before allowing direction to be steered by its member/s. (See Burnard, 1990, for group development and process.)

In summary, the role of facilitator involves the following:

- Encouraging the group to develop and maintain a trusting environment for facilitator and students.
- Encouraging openness and honesty which should help facilitate clarification of sexual attitudes, feelings and responses.

- Being sensitive to students' discomfort.
- Being as non-judgemental (as far as humanly possible) of others' beliefs. The facilitator has the potential to affect students' attitudes, values, feelings and knowledge, particularly if seen as a role model.
- Treating students as adults.
- Being comfortable with and able to express one's own sexuality.
- Always being attentive and receptive.
- Involving the students in the planning and direction the group should take.

Environment

The nature of the subject and its proposed style of facilitation demands consideration in respect of the environment. For group work which considers the subject of sexuality, a quiet, comfortable room is a necessity; nothing should be overheard from either inside or outside the room. Comfortable chairs should be used where possible, and students should be encouraged to sit in a circle (not behind desks). Allowing everybody to be seen and heard improves the 'feel' of the group. Refreshments in the room may also add to a more conducive atmosphere (Koch, 1985).

Small group work which involves up to 12 students provides a workable structure and environment. Using a small group set-up helps students to enhance their self-awareness, and increase personal and interpersonal contentment. It offers the students a sanctioned environment in which they can feel free to be open and honest about sexuality and sexual issues. Openness is a prerequisite to possible behaviour change and comfort for all those involved.

House rules

House rules or group guidelines are seen as a set of mutually agreed points. They form an agenda which is to be followed, and outline the expected behaviour of group members. The key phrase in this is that they are set by mutual agreement. The identification of house rules must be preceded by an overview of the programme's aims and objectives, together with the methods of facilitation. In other words, 'This is how we should behave', 'This is what we are going to look at', and 'This is how we are going to do it'. It is permissible at this early stage to point out that the aims and objectives may change. The group dynamics may cause a deviation from previously stated goals. Group needs are paramount, for conformity to predetermined rules, aims and objectives tend to stifle development and creativity. For this reason one should not attempt to generate a comprehensive list of rules that is set to cover all eventualities. See what happens, go with the flow.

Possible house rules may include the following.

- Participation – the collective sharing of ideas, thoughts and feelings, in response to group discussions and activities.
- Confidentiality – an agreement from all involved (including facilitator) that discussion about group material is not taken outside the group.
- Speaking in the first person – 'I think; I feel'.
- Passing – the ability to 'pass', or not take part in activities. Such passing is not questioned. However, the person passing should ask him/herself, 'Why am I passing?'
- Time out – the possibility to ask for a mutually agreed break.
- Attention – listen and give positive regard to what group members are saying.
- Closed group – once formed, the group does not allow extra members or observers to join.

A COURSE ON HUMAN SEXUALITY

The course is presented as a logical developmental progression. It is not submitted as a step-by-step guide to a course and what it should contain. It is a collection of activities which form a suggestive format for proceeding. This, in unison with the ideas expressed on group work and function, provides an important degree of flexibility. The activities cover a range of themes and are within the previously identified framework and premises. To recap these are:

Framework	*Premises*
Identification	*Holistic approach*
Densensitization	*Concept clarification*
Sensitization	*Values clarification*
Incorporation	*Nurse–patient relationship*
	Impact of illness on sexuality

The above areas will be identified by bold type in the subsequent activities, thus serving as a reminder to the structure and content of the programme. Additional activities could also be used from Chapter 6 which presents a range of case studies or scenarios which could be used as group activities or discussion points. The use of case scenarios demonstrates application to practice.

The nature of group development, coupled with the subject of sexuality, necessitates a gentle approach and introduction. An attempt to initiate deep, early discussion with a newly formed group could have lasting if not permanent and disastrous effects on students and facilitator. What is important in the opening session is 'scene setting'.

This means an explanation of what the course is about, together with participants' hopes and aspirations.

To initiate the group process there are a number of 'low-risk' activities available, which may or may not have a connection with sexuality. This is particularly important if the group is meeting for the first time. Attention needs to be brought to the group. Heather (1987) suggested that participants need a chance to 'off load' whatever is bothering them, or whatever they are concerned about elsewhere. She goes on to suggest the use of an activity called 'baggage dumping'. This is where participants are invited to form pairs, and to share the feelings and thoughts they were currently experiencing, or to share what happened to them at home that morning. There are other activities available, for example, Activity 5.

Activity 5: Ice breakers

Group members are invited in turn to respond to one or all of the following statements:

1. 'If I had a million pounds I would ...
2. 'Jim could fix it for me if he ...
3. 'If I were prime minister tomorrow I would ...
4. 'Last weekend I wish I ...
5. 'The thing I hate about this country is ...

Facilitator's note (time allowance 1 hour):

This opening 'ice breaker' allows the group members to relax; it is a form of 'getting to know you' activity which should be unthreatening. Group members should be encouraged to ask questions as people take it in turn to respond.

(More examples of activities can be found in Brandes and Phillips, 1984, Remocker and Storch, 1982).

There is no magic figure as to how many ice breakers or low-risk activities should be worked through before moving on to the primary subject. In practice, the decision is formed as much by experience as by intuition. In fact, the maxims 'if it feels right, do it', or 'feel the force' often apply and, surprisingly enough, work. Once what may be termed 'comfort level' has been reached, it is time to move on to examine the primary subject.

It is important at this point to remember that the depth or risk factor of activities is not held to be constant. As the attitude and feel of the group becomes more obvious, its life and well-being should be cultivated. To maintain the group members in 'high risk' activities can create a sober, more intense climate. Such activities are best used for short periods; it is more acceptable to have a varying degree of risk activities. The group will have peaks and troughs, the navigation of which should be guided by the group.

After a number of 'ice breakers' the activities should start to take a specific direction. This can be achieved by using an activity which is still non-threatening but which starts the ball rolling in raising awareness to the subject of sexuality. Activities 6, 7, 8 and 9 are possible examples.

Identification; concept clarification

Activity 6: Hopes and fears

Participants are asked to complete the following sentences:

1. What I hope to get out of the course on sexuality is . . .
2. My greatest worry about doing this course is . . .

Facilitator's note (time allowance 1 hour):

Students could be asked to respond to the above anonymously. The responses are then collected by the facilitator and written up on or read out to the group. Discussion takes place on the feelings and thoughts identified.

Alternative: as the facilitator reads out the cards, group members are invited to consider guessing who wrote the response. The writer need not admit to ownership.

Identification; concept clarification

Activity 7: What is this thing called sexuality anyway?

Group members are asked to consider possible answers to what they consider a definition of sexuality should involve.

Facilitator's note (time allowance 1.5 hours):

Participants are asked to consider their response to the above; this could involve working in groups, pairs or individually. Ideas are then displayed or discussed.

Identification; sensitization; concept clarification; values clarification

Activity 8: Art exhibition

Participants are split into two groups (a group of men and a group women, where possible). Each group is given a separate colle-tion of pictures, one set depicting men, another set depicting women. They are then asked to act as would-be art exhibitors. With the set of pictures, each respective group is asked to mount an exhibition, the main title of which is: 'The male, the female'. Participants are asked to give a subheading to the name of the exhibition, and if possible name the various pictures. When the display is complete, they should nominate a guide to take the whole group through the exhibition.

Facilitator's notes (time allowance 2 hours):

The pictures can be collected from various magazines, newspapers, etc, and should show men and women from a variety of settings, circum-stances and images. Enough room and display equipment should be made available. As the guide takes the group through the exhibition, it is important that the facilitator invites comments from the group.

Identification; densensitization; concept clarification; values clarification

Activity 9: Sexuality means to me . . .

Participants are asked to consider their responses to the following:

1. 'Sexuality is just about having good sex.'
2. 'Sexuality is a force driven by nature, and as such is nothing to do with the way you are brought up.'
3. 'Heterosexual sex is the only true form of sex.'
4. 'Sexuality is about going out for the evening and trying to pull a few birds.'
5. 'Everybody has sexual feelings.'
6. 'At what age do people realize they are straight, gay or lesbian?'
7. 'Men always want sex.'
8. 'When women say "no" they really mean "yes".'
9. 'Sexuality doesn't change with age.'
10. 'Sex is over-rated; love on the other hand isn't.'
11. 'Being a man means not showing your emotions.'
12. 'Women who are aggressive are usually labelled as feminists.'

Facilitator's note (time allowance 2 hours):

The above questions can be transferred to small cards and distributed around the group. Each person is then asked to read out the statement and give a response. Discussion takes place on the issues raised.

Alternative: some people may find it difficult to respond and voice an opinion. If the statements have been transferred onto postcards which are chosen because they depict a suggestion of sexuality, then the person can be asked to describe or interpret the meaning or impression the card produces, even to generate a story about the picture on the card.

Once a series of 'medium-risk' activities have been worked through, attention may be directed to examining 'high-risk' areas. The term 'high risk' is perhaps a little off-putting, and as such may activate the natural response mechanism of avoidance from students or facilitator. This avoidance or hesitation to enter into high-risk activities is a noteworthy issue, suggesting as it does the potential to open up emotive, deep and more personal issues surrounding sexuality. There are no hard and fast rules governing the decision to progress to this point. Whether a group moves into this area will depend on the skill, knowledge and awareness of the facilitator, together with the climate, development and security of the group. The following collection of activities demonstrate possible topic areas.

Identification; desensitization; sensitization; values clarification; nurse–patient relationship

Activity 10: Attraction

Participants are asked to sit in a circle and to turn to the person on their right and complete the following sentence.

- 'What a man would find attractive about you is . . .'

Facilitator's note (time allowance 1 hour):

It is important that the gender in the statement does not change. This may mean men saying it to men. After the exercise has gone round the group, the facilitator invites comments on what the activity felt like. Did people actually say what they wanted to say, or did they censor their response? What did it feel like to receive? And so on.

Alternatively, the gender in the statement could be changed, i.e. 'what a woman would find attractive about you is . . .'

Identification; desensitization; sensitization; values clarification

Activity 11: My sexuality

Participants are asked to take it in turns to complete the following.

- 'What I hate about my sexuality is . . .'
- 'What I like best about my sexuality is . . .'
- 'What makes it difficult to talk about sexual issues in a group like this is . . .'

Facilitator's note (time allowance 1.5 hours):

This activity may be carried out anonymously, with participants writing their responses on cards. The cards are collected and then read out; discussion should take place on issues raised.

Alternatively, the participants could take it in turns to verbally state their response to the three questions.

Identification; desensitization; sensitization; concept clarification; values clarification; nurse–patient relationship; impact of illness on sexuality

Activity 12: Unmentionables

Participants are invited to write anonymously on a piece of card what subject matter or issue they would not like to discuss within the group.

Facilitator's note (time allowance 5 mins or 1.5 hours):

Invariably the participants ask what will become of the information, and why do you want it? At this point it is important to state that they do not lose control over what will happen to their cards, the choice will be theirs.

On completion, the facilitator collects all the cards, they are then laid face down in the centre of the group, and the question is asked, 'What would you like to happen to these cards?' Students then might give a response; if they do not, the possibilities may be:

1. *Each one is read out and discussed.*
2. *Each one is read out and not discussed.*
3. *They are saved until a later date.*
4. *They are destroyed.*

Discussion takes place on the group's thoughts. If the group decides that the cards should be destroyed, this should be done in full view of the participants. If the cards are read out, it is crucial that a form of witch hunt does not ensue to find who said what. The responses may initiate discussion about taboo areas.

Identification; desensitization; sensitization; incorporation; holistic approach to patient care; concept clarification; values clarification; nurse–patient relationship; impact of illness on sexuality

Activity 13: Fancy that

What are your reactions, thoughts or feelings to the following scenarios?

1. What would you do if a patient (of opposite, or same sex) made a pass at you?
2. What would you do if you fancied a patient?
3. You are bed-bathing a man and he gets an erection; what would you do?
4. What do you do if a doctor makes a sexual pass at you?
5. Some patients think that male nurses are homosexuals. As a male nurse you think that this is affecting your relationship with the male patients. Even though you are not homosexual, what should you do?
6. Patients when nursed back to health regard nurses as 'angels of mercy' and as such look on them with a form of loving gratitude. Many men then start to incorporate such feelings into sexual arousal. This may manifest itself in blatant sexual invitations or pinching bottoms and stealing kisses. Is this a true state of affairs, and how should you react?
7. Male patients should be allowed time in the day to masturbate, especially young men on orthopaedic wards!
8. Old people have a reduced sexual appetite, so little consideration is needed for their sexual care.
9. It is not part of the nurse's role to get involved in discussing sexual matters with patients. Besides, it is too private.
10. The main reason why nurses do not get involved in the sexual side of patient care is the fact that they lack the necessary skills.

Facilitator's note (time allowance 2–3 hours or longer, depending on group response):

Participants may be split into small groups to discuss their thoughts and feelings about the above points. On reconvening, the facilitator may find a degree of group or individual conflict in values and views. If this is the case attempts should be made to move the students through the following processes.

1. *Identify the feeling you have, e.g. disgust, guilt, fear.*
2. *Identify the source of the feeling, e.g. parents, school, church.*
3. *Does your feeling affect personal or professional relationships?*
4. *If the answer to 3 is yes, is this due to lack of knowledge about the issue, or other factors?*
5. *Reassess your original value or point of view. Has it been affected, or has it:*

(a) *been strengthened?*

(b) *been modified?*

(c) *changed from the original value? If 'yes', to what value, and what factor caused the change?*

(d) *Affected the way you will look after patients in the future?*

Identification; desensitization; sensitization; concept clarification; values clarification

Activity 14: He's one of them

The following statements are distributed either individually or collectively to the participants. They are asked to consider whether they are true or false.

1. 'People are born homosexual.'
2. 'Homosexuality is a result of the way you were brought up.'
3. 'Gay men have a stronger relationship with their mothers than their fathers.'
4. 'Gays are responsible for AIDS; it is God's way of punishing them.'
5. 'It is impossible to live happily as a homosexual.'
6. 'Although I say now 'it won't make any difference to the way I care for him just because he's gay', in practice it would affect the way I care; I just could not help it.'
7. 'Gay men are basically scared of women, that is the root of the problem.'
8. 'Two gay men can have satisfying sex because they know what they each need.'
9. 'Homosexuality is on the increase because men are becoming more open about their feelings.'
10. 'I think we make a big thing about being gay in this country. After all, it is normal behaviour in other societies.'
11. 'Gay men should be able to adopt children.'

Facilitator's note (time allowance 2 hours):

It is important to establish the main themes that emerge on how participants see the concept of homosexuality, or being gay, and what prejudices participants hold about different sexual orientations and practices. If people have opposing views, split participants into groups and ask them to argue the opposite point of view. For example, those that believe 'homosexuals cannot live happily' should attempt to persuade another group that they can, and vice versa.

Identification; densensitization; sensitization; concept clarification; values clarification

Activity 15: Dykes

The following statements are distributed either individually or collectively to participants. They are asked to consider whether they are true or false.

1. 'Lesbians decry the most important aspect of being a woman, that is, to have children.'
2. 'Women who turn to lesbianism are just frightened of being dominated by men.'
3. 'Lesbians can't make proper love, because there's no penetration.'
4. 'I think it's right that lesbians should be able to have children.'
5. 'Those women who have lesbian affairs are not really lesbian, they're just looking for something different.'
6. 'Most lesbians are also strong feminists.'
7. 'I think if you really looked into it you would find there are more lesbian relationships than you thought. This is because it's not unusual for women to live together.'
8. 'Women turn to lesbianism because they can get a deeper form of affection and love than they can from a man.'
9. 'It's more acceptable to be a lesbian than it is to be a gay man.'
10. 'It wouldn't bother me if the female patient I was caring for was kissing and caressing her girlfriend during visiting time.'

Facilitator's note (time allowance 2 hours):

It is important to establish the main themes that emerge, and how participants see the concept of lesbianism. If people have opposing views, split participants into groups and ask them to argue the opposite point of view. For example, those that believe 'I think it's right that lesbians should be able to have children', should attempt to persuade another group that they should not, and vice versa.

Activities within this section can be supported with the use of video-taped material. There is an increasing number of purposefully produced films which can act as catalysts for discussion. The increase in the broadcasting of sex-related programmes on everyday television makes it possible to collect information to use in group activities. However, with this flourishing supply and use of sexual material it is possible to become too nonchalant about the whole subject. It is unwise to use video-tapes unless the feelings and emotions raised can be followed through and handled correctly. Over-exposure may lead to incorrect censorship of film material on the part of the facilitator. A useful safety net is to allow another colleague to see what you intend to use with the students, and gauge their reaction. As a facilitator, you should always ask the questions, 'Why am I showing this piece of video?' 'What purpose will it serve?' 'Are there underlying reasons?' 'Is the idea to agitate or to educate?'

Role-play is another useful technique to use, especially when exploring attitudes and prejudice to sexuality. For some students the idea of becoming involved in role-play fills them with abject panic, particularly when considering sexuality. Role-play is an approach that is best used when the group has matured, and the elements of trust and honesty are well established. If role-play is to be used then the idea of role-reversal is a useful method in helping students identify and work with varying attitudes and behaviours.

Identification; desensitization; sensitization; concept clarification; values clarification; nurse–patient relationship

Activity 16: Look at it this way

Participants are asked to consider an incident, encounter or recurring problem which involved differing attitudes or outright prejudice. A participant is then invited to describe the case. For example, 'Gay men are treated badly in hospital. Their lifestyle is seen as disgusting by some nurses and doctors.' An incident is then described in which participants take on the various roles.

Facilitator's notes (time allowance 1.5 hours):

If participants have difficulty in describing or enacting the situation, it may be useful to guide them through, giving participants certain roles and attitudes to act.

Once the role-play has been completed the participants should be asked for their thoughts and feelings about what it was like to play particular parts. If a participant holds strong attitudes, they could perhaps be persuaded to adopt the role they find difficult to understand. Seeing it from a different perspective may help in raising awareness.

On completing the role-play it is essential that participants are 'debriefed', or returned to their normal behaviour. The significance of the debriefing activity cannot be over-emphasized. It is therefore a prerequisite of any role-play, or for that matter any of the emotionally charged activities, that enough time is allowed. There are various methods available to debrief participants. One way is to invite each participant to express how they feel at that moment. The key component here is the emphasis on the present feelings (not thoughts), and not those experienced in the role-play. Participants should be asked to speak in the first person. For example, 'I feel more at ease with homosexuality now, because I've seen it from a different angle.' Another method of debriefing is to talk about future plans; what you are looking forward to during the weekend, for example. Further debriefing exercises can be found in Jaques' book *Learning in Groups* (1984).

EVALUATION

No course is complete without some form of evaluation. This is performed as much for the students as for the teacher and the organization. Evaluation could be built into the course as it progressed. For example, discussion after an activity, in which participants are allowed time to reflect on the experience and identify what they had learnt. Sometimes a round of each participant taking it in turns to complete the sentence, 'What I learnt today is . . .' or 'What I'm taking away from this session/workshop/course is ... ' Of course, it is also important to maintain the learning experience. Participants might like to work on activities in their own time. A useful remark to ask people to respond to is, 'The homework I'm giving myself today/this week/this month is ... '

The whole process of evaluation can be time consuming, and it may be necessary to allow an hour or so at the end of the sessions for the evaluation process. This time also allows for any 'unfinished business' to be brought up for discussion. The facilitator can ask, 'Does anybody have any final thoughts or feelings they'd like to discuss before we finish?' This usually starts the ball rolling. Finally, each participant is asked to say what they liked least and what they liked best about the course. It is important that any negative remarks come before the positive ones. Ending on a high note is as gratifying for the facilitator as it is for the participants.

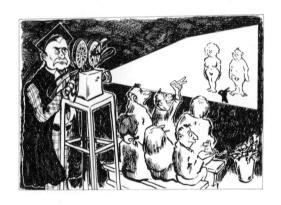

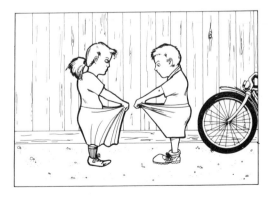

REFERENCES

Armstrong, K.F. and Wakeley, C. (1959) *Aids to Surgical Nursing*, 6th edn, Baillière Tindall & Cox, London.

Ashken, I.C. and Soddy, A.G. (1980) Study of pregnant school girls. *British Journal of Family Planning*, **6**, 77–82.

Bendall, E.R.D. and Raybould, E. (1970) *Basic Nursing*, 3rd edn, H.K. Lewis, London.

Brandes, D. and Phillips, R. (1984) *The Gamesters' Handbook, Vol. 2*, Hutchinson, London.

Bullough, V.L. and Seidl, I.A. (1987) Attitudes on sexuality in nursing texts today and yesterday. *Holistic Nursing Practice*, **1**(4), 84–92.

Burnard, P. (1990) *Teaching Interpersonal Skills. A Handbook of Experiential Learning for Health Professionals*, Chapman & Hall, London.

Bury, J.K. (1991) Teenage sexual behaviour and the impact of AIDS. *Health Education Journal*, **50**(1), 43–9.

Chapman, C.M. (1977) Concepts of professionalism. *Journal of Advanced Nursing*, **2**, 51–5.

Daily Express (1991) Having an adulterous affair. 10 July, 22–7.

Daily Mail (1991) Female forum. Why sex will become taboo again. 23 May, 36.

Department of Education and Science (1977) *Health Education in Schools*, HMSO, London.

Department of Education and Science (1986) *Children at School and Problems Related to AIDS*, HMSO, London.

Department of Education and Science (1987) *Sex Education at School*, No11/87, HMSO, London.

Donegan, J.B. (1975) Man – midwifery and the delicacy of the sexes, in *Remember the Ladies. New Perspectives on Women in American History* (ed. C.V. George), Syracuse University Press, New York.

Etzioni, A. (1969) *The Semi-Professions and Their Organizations*, Free Press, New York.

Family Planning Association (1984) *Sex Education in Schools*, FPA Fact Sheet D3, 3–4.

Frater, A. (1986) *Teenage Pregnancy Under-Sixteens 1969–1984, England and Wales*, Brook Advisory Centres Education and Publications Unit, Birmingham.

Galton, F. (1870) Cited by Flavia (1977) Victorian science and the genius of women. *Journal of Historical Ideas*, **38**, 261–80.

Gillick, V. (1986) The West Norfolk and Wisbech AHA and the DHSS (1986). *Appeals Case* (England) **112**.

Greaves, N.J. (1965) Sex education in colleges and departments of education. *Health Education Journal*, **24**(4), 171–7.

Hadfield, G. (1989) Sex: what Thatcher didn't want you to know. *The Sunday Times*, 17 September, 1.

Hansard (1980) *Publication of Information (Section 8)*. House of Commons, 30 June, Columns 369–70.

Heather, B. (1987) *Sharing: A Handbook for Those Involved in Training in Personal Relationships and Sexuality*, FPA Education Unit, London.

Hogan, R. (1980) *Human Sexuality: A Nursing Perspective*, Appleton-Century-Crofts, New York.

Humphries, S. (1988) *A Secret World of Sex. Forbidden Fruit: The British Experience 1900–1950*, Sidgwick & Jackson, London.

The Independent (1991) Sex education should start at five say MPS, 7 November, 7.

Jackson, D. (1989) Sex education in Halton secondary school. *Health Visitor*, July, **62**, 219–21.

Jaques, D. (1984) *Learning in Groups*, Croom Helm, London.

Johnson, A.M., Wadsworth, J., Wellings, K. *et al.* (1992) Sexual lifestyles and HIV risk. *Nature*, **360**, 3 December, 410–12.

Jones, E.F., Forrest, J.D. and Goldman, N. (1985) Teenage pregnancy in developed countries: determinants and policy implications. *Family Planning Perspectives*, **17**, 53–63.

Kautz, D.D. *et al.* (1990) Using research to identify why nurses do not meet established sexuality nursing care standards. *Journal of Nursing Quality Assurance*, **4**(3), 68–78.

Kilroy-Silk, R. (1992) *Sex Education*, BBC Television, 15 April.

Koch, J.J. (1985) Psychotherapeutic techniques and methods applied in teaching human sexuality. *Journal of Nursing Education*, **8**, 346–9.

Llewellyn-Jones, D. (1991) *Everyman*, 3rd edn, Oxford University Press, Oxford.

Local Government Act (1988) *Section 28*, HMSO, London.

Ludlow, E.A. and Bagwell, M. (1983) Faculty and students confront sexuality. *Journal of Nursing Education*, **22**(4), 161–4.

Mandetta, A.F. and Woods, N.F. (1974) Learning about human sexuality – a course model. *Nursing Outlook*, **22**, 525–7.

Masters, W.H. and Johnson, V.E. (1966) *Human Sexual Response*, Little, Brown, Boston.

McMahon, K. (1990) The cosmopolitan ideology and the management of desire. *The Journal of Sex Research*, **27**(3), 381–96.

Meredith, L. (1984) Some thoughts on teaching student nurses human sexuality. *Lamp*, **41**(2), 21–2.

Miller, S. (1984) Recognizing the sexual health care needs of hospitalized patients. *Canadian Nurse*, **80**(3), 43–6, 49.

Ministry of Education (1957) *Health Education Pamphlet 31*, HMSO, London.

Morry van Ments (1983) *The Effective Use of Role Play. A Handbook for Teachers and Trainers*, Kogan Page, London.

National Curriculum Council (1991) *Science in the National Curriculum, Health Education 5. Key Stages 1–4*, NCC, York.

Nursing Times (1993) Sex education cuts threaten health aim. *Nursing Times*, **89**(1), 8.

OPCS Monitor (1989) *Office of Population Census and Surveys. Legal Abortions*, OPCS, London.

Payne, T. (1976) Sexuality of nurses: correlations of knowledge, attitudes and behaviour. *Nursing Research*, **25**, 286–92.

Pearce, E. (1960) *The General Textbook of Nursing*, 5th edn, Faber & Faber, London.

Quinn-Krach, P. and van Hoozer, H. (1988) Sexuality of the aged and the attitudes and knowledge of nursing students. *Journal of Nursing Education*, **27**(8), 359–63.

Rea, N. (1974) in Nazer, I.R. (1976) *Sex Education in Schools: Proceedings of an Expert Group Meeting.* International Planned Parenthood Federation, Middle East and North Africa Region.

Remocker, A.J. and Storch, E.T. (1982) *Action Speaks Louder. A Handbook of Non-Verbal Group Techniques*, Churchill Livingstone, Edinburgh.

Robb, I.H. (1907) *Nursing: Its Principles and Practice for Hospital and Private Use*, J.A. Carreth, Toronto, p. 401.

Roche, A.F. (1979) Secular trends in human growth, maturation and development. *Monogr. Sociological Research and Child Development*, **44**, 3–4.

Roper, N., Logan, W.W. and Tierney, A.J. (1980) *The Elements of Nursing*, Churchill Livingstone, Edinburgh.

Savage, J. (1987) *Nurses, Gender and Sexuality*. Nursing Today Series, Heinemann Nursing, London.

Sayer, J. and Semple, J. (1958) *Aids to Male Genito-Urinary Nursing*, 3rd edn, Baillière Tindall & Cox, Eastbourne.

Scott, L. and Thomson, R. (1992) School sex education: More a patchwork than a pattern. *Health Education Journal*, **51**(3), 132–5.

Tanner, J.M. (1968) Earlier maturation in man. *Scientific America*, **218**(1), 21–7.

Thomas, A.P. (1986) A survey of sex education in a Welsh local education authority. Unpublished MEd thesis, University of Wales, Cardiff.

Thomas, B. (1990) Working out sexuality. *Nursing Times*, **86**, 41–3.

Today (1993) 12–15 January.

Tucker, A. and Prout, M. (1937) Sex education in schools: an experiment in elementary instruction, in Greaves, N.J. (1965) Sex education in colleges and departments of education. *Health Education Journal*, **24**(4), 171–7.

Ustinov, P.(1992) *Dear Me*, Mandarin, London.

Vincent, C.E. (1968) Report on institute held at the behavioural science center of Bowman Gray School of Medicine of Wake Forest College, Winston-Salem, N.C., in Walker, E.G. (1971) Study of sexuality in the nursing curriculum. *Nursing Forum*, **10**(1), 18–30.

Waltley, L.A. (1983) Male physicians and female health and sexuality in 19th century English and American society. *Journal of Advanced Nursing*, **8**, 423–8.

Waterhouse, J. and Metcalfe, M. (1991) Attitudes towards nurses discussing sexual concerns with patients. *Journal of Advanced Nursing*, **16**, 1048–54.

Webb, C. and Wilson-Barnett, J. (1983) Self-concept, social support and hysterectomy. *International Journal of Nursing Studies*, **20**(2), 97–107.

Webb, C. (1985) Teaching sexuality in the curriculum. *Senior Nurse*, **3**(5), 10–12.

Webb, C. (1987) Sexuality: sexual healing. *Nursing Times*, **83**(32), 28–30.

White Paper (1992) *The Health of the Nation: A Strategy for Health in England*. Department of Health, HMSO, London.

Appendix A

GLOSSARY

Abortion	A procedure which terminates pregnancy; it may be therapeutic or spontaneous
Abstinence	Not engaging in sexual intercourse
Adultery	Having sexual intercourse outside the marriage
AIDS	Acquired immune deficiency syndrome
Amenorrhoea	The absence of menstruation (periods)
Anal sex (intercourse)	The penis is placed in the anus
Androgen	The male hormone
Annilingus	The tongue is moved around the anus
Aphrodisiacs	A substance, food, animal or mineral, which when taken is said to increase the sex drive
Asexual	Not engaging in sexual activity
Bestiality (zoophilia)	Sexual interest in animals
Bigamy	Going through with a marriage while already married
Bisexuality	A sexual interest in both males and females
Brothel	A house which supports prostitution, male or female
Celibacy	No sexual activity
Cervix	The narrow part of the uterus
Circumcision	The surgical removal of the foreskin which covers the head of the penis
Clitoris	A sensitive organ which is found just above the urethral opening near the vaginal entrance
Coitus	Sexual intercourse; joining together of male and female organs; making love
Coitus interruptus	See withdrawal

Coming out	A term used to describe a homosexual person making his/her sexual orientation known to heterosexual people
Condom	A form of birth control made of latex, it is used to cover the penis during intercourse. This stops sperm entering the vagina. They are also available for women
Coprophilia	Erotic fascination with faeces
Cunnilingus	Using the tongue around the vagina
Curse	Menstruation
Dildo	An artificial penis
Dykes	Slang word for female homosexuals
Dysmenorrhoea	Painful menstruation
Dyspareunia	Painful intercourse
Ejaculation	The expelling of semen from the male genitals on reaching orgasm
Erection	When the male genital fills with blood, causing the penis to rise
Erotic	Give sexual pleasure
Erogenous zones	Areas on the body which when stimulated produce sensual satisfacton, e.g. anus, mouth, genitals
Eunuch	Castrated man, i.e. loss of testes
Exhibitionism	Exposing genitals to people who are unsuspecting
Fellatio	Using the mouth to stimulate the male genitalia
Femidom	Female condom made from latex
Fetishism	Using objects for sexual stimulation
Flagellation	Flogging as a means of sexual stimulation
Foreplay	Activities which start to arouse sexual interest, e.g. kissing, touching
Fornicating	Sexual intercourse
Fuck	Slang term for sexual intercourse
Gay	A term used to describe a person as homosexual
Gender	A person's biological sex – male or female
Genitals	Male or female sex organs
Hermaphrodite	Person has a condition at birth when the sex organs of both the male and female are present
Heterosexual	Attraction to opposite sex
Homophobia	Dislike or fear of homosexuals
Homosexuality	Sexual interest in people of the same sex

Human immuno-deficiency virus (HIV)	Virus which may cause AIDS
Hysterectomy	Surgical removal of the uterus
Impotence	Inability to attain and maintain penile erection
Impotent	Unable to reach sexual orgasm
Incest	Sexual contact of people who are related by blood or marriage, excluding spouses
Intercourse	Action of joining together of male and female genitals; making love
Inversion	People who have contrary sexual feelings (Freud)
Kelismaphilia	Using enemas for sexual stimulation
Lesbianism	Female to female sexual attraction
Libido	Sexual drive; the desire to have sex activity
Masturbation	Individual or mutual stimulation of sexual organs
Menarche	The first menstrual period
Menses	The periodic flow of blood during menstruation
Menstrual cycle	Refers to the periodic release of an ovum and the shedding of cells or lining of the uterus if fertilization has not taken place
Menstruation	Blood from the uterus, usually every month, for an average of five days' duration
Monogamous	Having one sex partner
Narcissism	Love for or of self
Nymphomania	Over-active sexual behaviour in women
Oedipus	Freudian theory of child's erotic attachment to its mother
Oral sex	Stimulating the genitals with the mouth
Orgasm	Reaching a peak of sexual stimulation, with ejaculation of semen in the male
Ovum	The female egg
Paedophilia	Sexual activity with children
Pederasty	Sexual involvement between men and boys
Penis	Male sex organ
Perversion	Abnormal behaviour or liking; usually refers to sexual activity other than normal
Phallus	Relating to the male genitalia, usually erect
Pimp	A man who offers to look after and arrange clients for a female prostitute
Platonic	Non-erotic love
Pornography	Material with the primary intention of causing sexual arousal

Premature ejaculation	The inability to consciously control semen
Prostitution	Sexual activity by males or females for money
Pubic hair	The growth of hair in the genital area
Pulling a bird	Forming a relationship (or getting a date) with a women; has sexual connotations
Sadism	Sexual pleasure from watching or inflicting cruelty
Sadomasochism	Giving or receiving pain as sexual pleasure
Satyriasis	Over-active sexual behaviour in men
Semen	The sperm, and prostatic secretions
Sensate focus	Touching and stroking of partner without engaging in sexual activity
Sex education	Providing information about sexual matters
Sexual arousal	Excitement brought on by another person or object; being 'turned on'
Sexual desire	Factors which promote a person to engage in sexual relationships
Smegma	A cheese-like substance produced by glands in the head of the penis
Sodomy	Anal intercourse usually between males
Sperm	The male cells of reproduction
Stereotype	A way of collectively thinking or labelling a person because of their behaviour or attitude
Transsexuals	People who believe they are the opposite to their biological sex
Transvestism	Wearing the clothes of the opposite sex for sexual excitement
Uterus	Muscular organ in which eggs are implanted and the fetus develops until it is expelled
Vagina	A muscular canal which is the common passage for intercourse and birth of the baby
Vibrator	A battery-operated device to be used for sexual stimulation
Voyeurism	Deriving sexual gratification from secretly observing sexual activities
Vulva	External female sex organs
Wanking	See masturbation
Withdrawal	The method of birth control which involves the removal of the penis from the vagina before ejaculation
Zoophilia	See bestiality

Glossary of colloquialisms and euphemisms

The male sex organ

- penis
- knob
- dick
- John Thomas
- member
- shaft
- Jimmy
- Willy
- love truncheon
- meat and two veg.
- old man
- plonker
- tool

The female sex organ

- vagina
- down below
- under-carriage
- foof
- cunt
- twat
- Mary
- Jenny May
- crack
- fanny
- pussy
- clit
- beaver

Sexual intercourse

- screwing
- bonking
- fucking
- on the nest
- shafting
- knee trembler
- leg-over
- getting laid
- getting it together
- roll in the hay

Condoms

- French letter
- safe
- Durex
- sheath

Appendix B

USEFUL ADDRESSES

Albany Trust. 24 Chester Square, London SW1W 9HS. Tel: 071-730 5871.
  (Individual or group counselling for relationship or psychosexual problems.)
ARMS (Action for Research into Multiple Sclerosis). Operates a 24-hour telephone counselling service on 071-222 3123.
BACUP (British Association of Cancer United Patients). 121/123 Charterhouse Street, London EC1M 6AA. Tel: 071-608 1661.
  (Cancer information and support.)
Beaumont Society. PO Box 3084, London WC1V 3XX.
  (Provides counselling for transvestites.)
Body Positive. 51b Philbeach Gardens, London SW5 9EB. Tel: 071-373 9124.
  (Help for those diagnosed HIV-positive.)
Breast Care and Mastectomy Association. 26a Harrison Street, Off Gray's Inn Road, Kings Cross, London WC1H 8JG. Tel: 071-837 0908.
Bristol Cancer Help Centre, Grove House, Cornwallis Grove, Clifton, Bristol BS8 4PG. Tel: 0272 743216.
British Colostomy Association. 13–15 Station Road, Reading, Berkshire RG1 1LB. Tel: 0734 391537.
Brook Advisory Centres. 153 East Street, London SE17 2SD. Tel: 071-708 1390.
Childline. Tel: 0800 1111.
Disabled Living Foundation (DLF). 380–84 Harrow Road, London W9 2HU. Tel: 071-289 6111.
Family Planning Association (FPA). Margaret Pyke House, 27–35 Mortimer Street, London W1A 4QW. Tel: 071-636 7866.
Gay Men's Disabled Group. c/o Gays the Word, 66 Marchmount Street, London WC1 1AB.

Gemma. BM Box 5700, London WC1V 6XX. An organization for homosexual women who are disabled.

GLAD (Greater London Association for the Disabled). 336 Brixton Road, London SW9 7AA. Tel: 071-274 0107.

Health Education Authority. Hamilton House, Mabledon Place, London WC1H 9TX. Tel: 071-383 3833.

Hysterectomy Support Group. Ann Webb, 1 Henryson Road, Brockley, London SE4 1HL. Tel: 081-690 5987.

Ileostomy Association. Amblehurst House, Black Scotch Lane, Mansfield, Nottinghamshire NG18 4PF. Tel: 0623 28099.

Incest Crisis Line. Tel: 081-890 4732/422 5100.

Lesbian and Gay Switchboard. Tel: 071-837 7324.

Let's Face It. Christine Piff, 10 Wood End, Crowthorne, Berks RG11 6DG. Tel: 0344 774405.
(Provides a support network for people with facial handicap).

Relate (National Marriage Guidance). Tel: 0788 73241, for nearest branch.

Spastics Society. 16 Fitzroy Square, London W1. Tel: 071-387 9571.

Spinal Injuries Association. Yeoman House, 76 St James's Lane, London N10 3DF. Tel: 081-444 2121.

SPOD (Association to Aid the Sexual and Personal Relationships of People with a Disability). 286 Camden Road, London N70 BJ. Tel: 071-607 8851.

The Stroke Association. CHSA House, Whitecross Street, London EC1Y 8JJ. Tel: 071-490 7999.

Terence Higgins Trust. BM AIDS, London WC1N 3XX. Tel: 071-242 1010.

Urostomy Association. 'Buckland', Beaumont Park, Danbury, Essex CM3 4DE. Tel: 024-541 4294.

Welsh AIDS Helpline. PO Box 348, Cardiff CF1 4XL. Tel: 0222 223443.

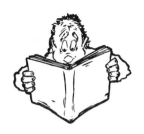

Index

Page numbers appearing in **bold** refer to figures.